# INSTRUCTION MANUAL IN
# OBSTETRICS

VOLUME ONE

# INSTRUCTION MANUAL IN
# OBSTETRICS

## DR. LAMIAA MOUSA AL-MADANY

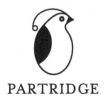

PARTRIDGE

Library of Congress Control Number:    2017953954
ISBN:          Hardcover          978-1-5437-4252-7
               Softcover          978-1-5437-4251-0
               eBook              978-1-5437-4250-3

Print information available on the last page.

**To order additional copies of this book, contact**
Toll Free 800 101 2657 (Singapore)
Toll Free 1 800 81 7340 (Malaysia)
orders.singapore@partridgepublishing.com

www.partridgepublishing.com/singapore

# Table of Contents

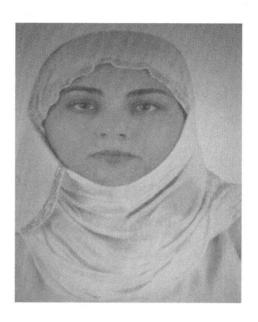

**Dr: Lamiaa   Mousa   AL-Madany**

**Consultant Obstetric and Gynecology**
Arab Board in Obstetric and Gynecology
MSC Quality & Safety in Healthcare Management
Certified Professional in Health & Hospital Administration
Member in Saudi Obstetric & Gynecological Society
Member of the European Society Of
Contraception And Reproductive Health
Member in Egyption Society of Maternal Fetal Medicine
Member in Saudi Osteoporosis Society
Member in Saudi Cancer Foundation

# Instruction Manual in Obstetrics

## Why to read this book

Evidence base knowledge is the most important factor to develop up to date standard of practice.

The aim of this book is to summarize the practical knowledge needed by an obstetrician and gynecologist to manage the patient in an out-patient clinic and labour room.

The information in this book is kept as headline which the physician will read, this information will not cover all the topic it will be the most important headline which is summarized in flow charts.

The aim of the flow chart is to carry out the short way which activate the physician's brain to remember by creating a brain map image.

## Who is this book for?

If you can answer, "yes" to any of these:

1. Are you physician treating a female in obstetric and gynecology clinic?
2. Do you want to learn, understand, remember, and apply important updated evidence base information so you can treat your patient with high level of trust?
3. Do you want to pass the board exam, and learn to be a better obstetrician and gynecologist?

4. Do you prefer stimulating attractive challenging way of learning?

**Then this book is for you.**

## After finishing this book you will be able to

1. Earn more self-confidence
2. Manage your patient in better way
3. earn your peer respect
4. stand in solid ground standing for medico legal cases
5. Strong base in teaching your junior
6. Gain more confidants to inter the board examination

# Section I Instruction manual in Obstetric Clinic

# 1 Follow up of normal pregnancy

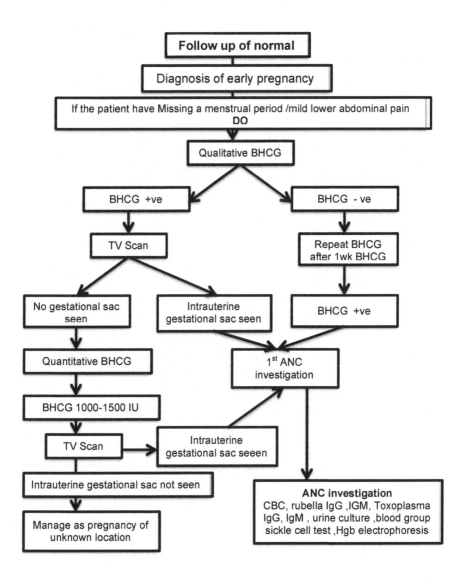

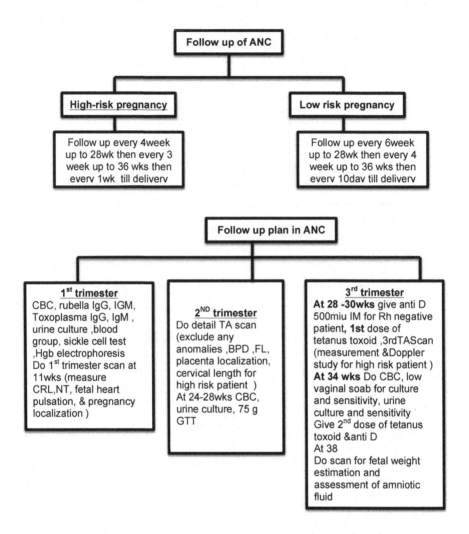

**Follow up of ANC**

**High-risk pregnancy**

Follow up every 4week up to 28wk then every 3 week up to 36 wks then every 1wk till delivery

**Low risk pregnancy**

Follow up every 6week up to 28wk then every 4 week up to 36 wks then every 10day till delivery

**Follow up plan in ANC**

**1st trimester**
CBC, rubella IgG, IGM, Toxoplasma IgG, IgM , urine culture ,blood group, sickle cell test ,Hgb electrophoresis
Do 1st trimester scan at 11wks (measure CRL,NT, fetal heart pulsation, & pregnancy localization )

**2ND trimester**
Do detail TA scan (exclude any anomalies ,BPD ,FL, placenta localization, cervical length for high risk patient )
At 24-28wks CBC, urine culture, 75 g GTT

**3rd trimester**
**At 28 -30wks** give anti D 500miu IM for Rh negative patient, **1st** dose of tetanus toxoid ,3rdTAScan (measurement &Doppler study for high risk patient )
**At 34 wks** Do CBC, low vaginal soab for culture and sensitivity, urine culture and sensitivity
Give 2nd dose of tetanus toxoid &anti D
At 38
Do scan for fetal weight estimation and assessment of amniotic fluid

# 2   First trimester vaginal bleeding

First trimester vaginal bleeding

History of
1.last menstrual period
2.past obstetric history of abortion
3.past history of ectopic pregnancy
4.past history of PID
5.history of coagulation disorder

Examination
1.scheck vital sign
2.examin the abdomen for softness
tenderness, rebound tenderness
3.speculum to examine any sign of injury,
source of bleeding any abnormality in the
cervix or bleeding from uterus

Lower abdominal pain, Open cervix with vaginal bleeding, and product of conception.

+/-Lower abdominal pain, close cervix with minimal vaginal bleeding

Local cause vaginal or cervical cause

# 2.1 Management &treatment of first trimester vaginal bleeding

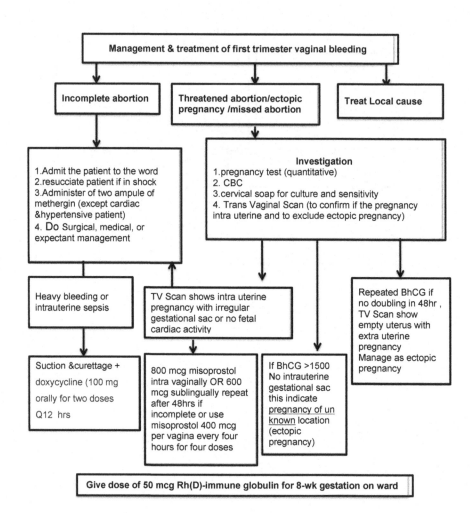

**Management & treatment of first trimester vaginal bleeding**

**Incomplete abortion**

**Threatened abortion/ectopic pregnancy /missed abortion**

**Treat Local cause**

1.Admit the patient to the word
2.resucciate patient if in shock
3.Administer of two ampule of methergin (except cardiac &hypertensive patient)
4. Do Surgical, medical, or expectant management

**Investigation**
1.pregnancy test (quantitative)
2. CBC
3.cervical soap for culture and sensitivity
4. Trans Vaginal Scan (to confirm if the pregnancy intra uterine and to exclude ectopic pregnancy)

Heavy bleeding or intrauterine sepsis

TV Scan shows intra uterine pregnancy with irregular gestational sac or no fetal cardiac activity

Repeated BhCG if no doubling in 48hr , TV Scan show empty uterus with extra uterine pregnancy Manage as ectopic pregnancy

Suction &curettage + doxycycline (100 mg orally for two doses Q12 hrs

800 mcg misoprostol intra vaginally OR 600 mcg sublingually repeat after 48hrs if incomplete or use misoprostol 400 mcg per vagina every four hours for four doses

If BhCG >1500 No intrauterine gestational sac this indicate pregnancy of un known location (ectopic pregnancy)

**Give dose of 50 mcg Rh(D)-immune globulin for 8-wk gestation on ward**

# 2.2 Vaginal bleeding with positive pregnancy test

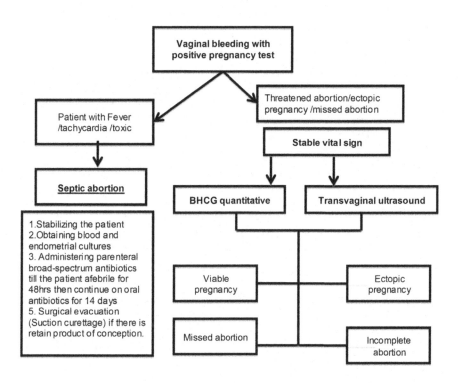

# 2.3   Ultrasound with vaginal bleeding

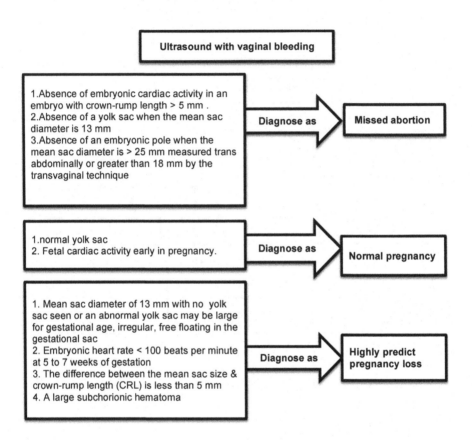

Ultrasound with vaginal bleeding

1.Absence of embryonic cardiac activity in an embryo with crown-rump length > 5 mm .
2.Absence of a yolk sac when the mean sac diameter is 13 mm
3.Absence of an embryonic pole when the mean sac diameter is > 25 mm measured trans abdominally or greater than 18 mm by the transvaginal technique

Diagnose as → Missed abortion

1.normal yolk sac
2. Fetal cardiac activity early in pregnancy.

Diagnose as → Normal pregnancy

1. Mean sac diameter of 13 mm with no yolk sac seen or an abnormal yolk sac may be large for gestational age, irregular, free floating in the gestational sac
2. Embryonic heart rate < 100 beats per minute at 5 to 7 weeks of gestation
3. The difference between the mean sac size & crown-rump length (CRL) is less than 5 mm
4. A large subchorionic hematoma

Diagnose as → Highly predict pregnancy loss

# 2.4   Septic abortion

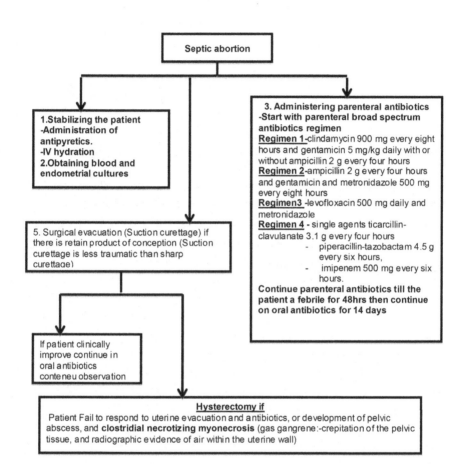

**Septic abortion**

**1.Stabilizing the patient**
-Administration of antipyretics.
-IV hydration
**2.Obtaining blood and endometrial cultures**

**3. Administering parenteral antibiotics**
-Start with parenteral broad spectrum antibiotics regimen
**Regimen 1-**clindamycin 900 mg every eight hours and gentamicin 5 mg/kg daily with or without ampicillin 2 g every four hours
**Regimen 2**-ampicillin 2 g every four hours and gentamicin and metronidazole 500 mg every eight hours
**Regimen3** -levofloxacin 500 mg daily and metronidazole
**Regimen 4** - single agents ticarcillin-clavulanate 3.1 g every four hours
-    piperacillin-tazobactam 4.5 g every six hours,
-    imipenem 500 mg every six hours.
**Continue parenteral antibiotics till the patient a febrile for 48hrs then continue on oral antibiotics for 14 days**

5. Surgical evacuation (Suction curettage) if there is retain product of conception (Suction curettage is less traumatic than sharp curettage)

If patient clinically improve continue in oral antibiotics conteneu observation

**Hysterectomy if**
 Patient Fail to respond to uterine evacuation and antibiotics, or development of pelvic abscess, and **clostridial necrotizing myonecrosis** (gas gangrene:-crepitation of the pelvic tissue, and radiographic evidence of air within the uterine wall)

# 3   Venous thromboprophylactic

*All women should undergo a documented of risk factors for VTE in early pregnancy or pre-pregnancy. Risk assessment should be repeated if the woman is* **admitted to hospital** *for any reason or develops other intercurrent problems. Risk assessment should be repeated again* **intrapartum** *or* **immediately postpartum.**

# 3.1 Risk assessment od venous thromboembolism in antenatal patient

## High Risk Factor will score 4
1.Any previous VTE except a single event related to major surgery.
2.Pregnant women with APS.
3.Pregnant women with prior VTE
4.Pregnant women with prior arterial thrombosis.
5.Pregnant women with previous VTE associated with antithrombin deficiency.

## Mild Risk Factor will score 1:
1.Obesity (BMI > 30 kg / m2.
2.Age > 35
3.Parity ≥ 3.
4.Smoker.
5.Gross varicose veins.
6.Current pre-eclampsia.
7.Immobility, e.g. paraplegia, PGP.
8.Family history of unprovoked or estrogen-
9.provoked VTE in first degree relative.
10.Family history of unprovoked or estrogen-
11.provoked VTE in first degree relative.
12.Low-risk thrombobophilia.
13Multiple pregnancies IVF/ART.

## Intermediate Risk Factor will Score 3:

1.Hospital admission.
2.Single previous VTE related to major surgery.
3.High Risk thrombophilia + NO VTE.
4.Homozygous factor V Leiden.
5.Compound hetrozygote protein C deficiency.
6.Compound hetrozygote protein S deficiency.

## Medical Comorbidities:
1.Patient with cancer.
2.Patient with heart failure.
3.Patient with IBD.
4.Patient with active SLE.
5.Patient with inflammatory polyarthropathy.
6.Patient with nephrotic syndrome.
7.Patient with Type I DM with nephropathy.
8.Patient with sickle cell disease, current IVDU.
9.Patient with current IVDU.
10.Patient with any surgical procedure e.g appendectomy.

## Transient Risk Factors: will receive LMWH as long the transient risk factor excess:

1.Patient with dehydration hyperemesis.
2.Patient with ovarian hyper stimulation syndrome.

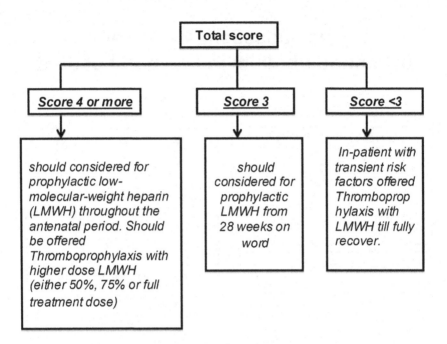

```
                    ┌──────────────┐
                    │  Total score │
                    └──────┬───────┘
        ┌──────────────────┼──────────────────┐
```

| Score 4 or more | Score 3 | Score <3 |

| should considered for prophylactic low-molecular-weight heparin (LMWH) throughout the antenatal period. Should be offered Thromboprophylaxis with higher dose LMWH (either 50%, 75% or full treatment dose) | should considered for prophylactic LMWH from 28 weeks on word | In-patient with transient risk factors offered Thromboprop hylaxis with LMWH till fully recover. |

**ANTENATAL PROPHYLACTIC DOSE OF LMWH:**
Weight < 50 kg, give 20 mg enoxaparin daily.
Weight > 50-90 kg, give 40 mg enoxaparin daily.
Weight 91-130 kg, give 60 mg enoxaparin daily.
Weight 131-70 kg, give 80 mg enoxaparin daily.
Weight > 170 kg, give 6 mg /kg/day enoxaparin daily.

10

# 3.2 Risk assessment od venous thromboembolism in postenatal patient

**High Risk Factor will score 4**

1.Any previous VTE except a single event related to major surgery.
2.Patient with anyone requiring Antenatal LMWH
3.Patient with high risk thrombophilia homozygous factor V Leiden.
4.Patient with compound hetrozygote protein C or S deficiency.
5.Low Risk thrombophilia + family history of thromboembolic events.

**Mild Risk Factor will score 1:**

1.Obesity (BMI > 30 kg / m2.
2.Age > 35
3.Parity ≥ 3.
4.Patient with Elective Cesarean Section.
5.Gross varicose veins.
6.Current pre-eclampsia.
7.Immobility, e.g. paraplegia, PGP.
8.Family history of unprovoked or estrogen-9.provoked VTE in first-degree relative.
10.Low-risk thromphobophilia.
11.Patient with long distance travel.
12.Patient with multiple pregnancies.
13.Patient with pre-term delivery, in this pregnancy (<37+0 weeks).
14.Patient with stillbirth in this pregnancy.
15.Patient with Mid-cavity rotational or operative delivery.
16.Multiple pregnancies IVF/ART.
17.Patient with prolonged labour (> 24 hours).
18.Patient with PPH > 1 liter or blood transfusion.

**Intermediate Risk Factor will Score 3:**

1. Cesarean Section in labour.
2.BMI ≥ 40 kg / m2.
3.Readmission or prolonged admission (≥ 3 days) in the puerperium.
4.Any surgical procedure in the puerperium except immediate repair of the perineum.
5.Medical Comorbidities:
6.Patient with cancer.
7.Patient with heart failure.
8.Patient with IBD.
9.Patient with active SLE
10.Patient with inflammatory polyarthropathy.
11.Patient with nephrotic syndrome.
12.Patient with Type I DM with nephropathy
13.Patient with sickle cell disease, current IVDU        14.Patient with current IVDU.
15Patient with any surgical procedure e.g. appendectomy.

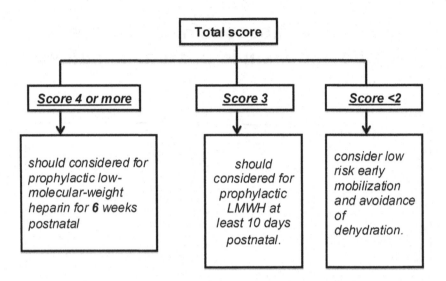

---

**ANTENATAL PROPHYLACTIC DOSE OF LMWH:**
Weight < 50 kg, give 20 mg enoxaparin daily.
Weight > 50-90 kg, give 40 mg enoxaparin daily.
Weight 91-130 kg, give 60 mg enoxaparin daily.
Weight 131-70 kg, give 80 mg enoxaparin daily.
Weight > 170 kg, give 6 mg /kg/day enoxaparin daily.

# 4 Thrombocytopenia during pregnancy

> **Thrombocytopenia during pregnancy**

**Thrombocytopenia during pregnancy**

- 1.Gestational thrombocytopenia
- 2.TTP/HUS
- 3.Drug-induced ITTP
- 4.Antiphospholipid syndrome thrombocytopenia
- 4.ITTP Immune thrombocytopenic purpura

**Antenatal**
- Forceps and vacuum assisted delivery are relatively contraindicated, if it is indicated use forceps rather than vacuum assisted deliver
-Cesarean delivery reserved only for standard obstetrical indications

**Post natal**
Antiplatelet drugs (eg, aspirin, nonsteroidal antiinflammatory drugs) should be avoided postpartum in women with thrombocytopenia.

# 4.1 Management of patient with ITTP

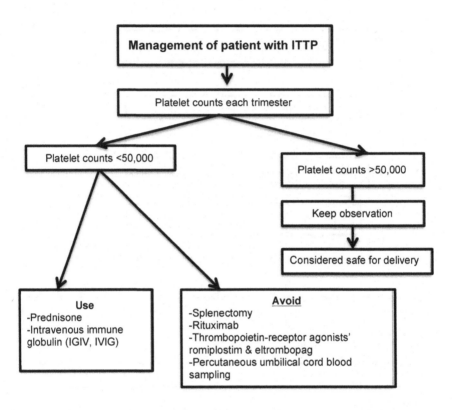

# 4.2 Causes of Thrombocytopenia during pregnancy

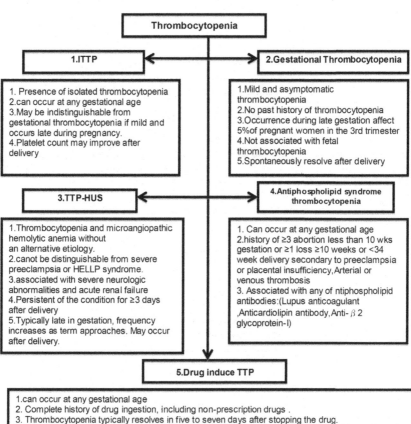

**Thrombocytopenia**

**1.ITTP**

1. Presence of isolated thrombocytopenia
2. can occur at any gestational age
3. May be indistinguishable from gestational thrombocytopenia if mild and occurs late during pregnancy.
4. Platelet count may improve after delivery

**2.Gestational Thrombocytopenia**

1. Mild and asymptomatic thrombocytopenia
2. No past history of thrombocytopenia
3. Occurrence during late gestation affect 5%of pregnant women in the 3rd trimester
4. Not associated with fetal thrombocytopenia
5. Spontaneously resolve after delivery

**3.TTP-HUS**

1. Thrombocytopenia and microangiopathic hemolytic anemia without an alternative etiology.
2. canot be distinguishable from severe preeclampsia or HELLP syndrome.
3. associated with severe neurologic abnormalities and acute renal failure
4. Persistent of the condition for ≥3 days after delivery
5. Typically late in gestation, frequency increases as term approaches. May occur after delivery.

**4.Antiphospholipid syndrome thrombocytopenia**

1. Can occur at any gestational age
2. history of ≥3 abortion less than 10 wks gestation or ≥1 loss ≥10 weeks or <34 week delivery secondary to preeclampsia or placental insufficiency, Arterial or venous thrombosis
3. Associated with any of ntiphospholipid antibodies:(Lupus anticoagulant ,Anticardiolipin antibody, Anti-$\beta$2 glycoprotein-I)

**5.Drug induce TTP**

1. can occur at any gestational age
2. Complete history of drug ingestion, including non-prescription drugs .
3. Thrombocytopenia typically resolves in five to seven days after stopping the drug.
4. Heparin-induced thrombocytopenia platelet drop by 50% of platelet count for patient begun heparin within previous 5 to 10 days.
5. ELISA assay for heparin-dependent antibodies is sensitive; measurement of heparin-induced platelet serotonin release is more specific.

# 5 Anemia in pregnancy

## 5.1 Definition of Anemia in pregnancy

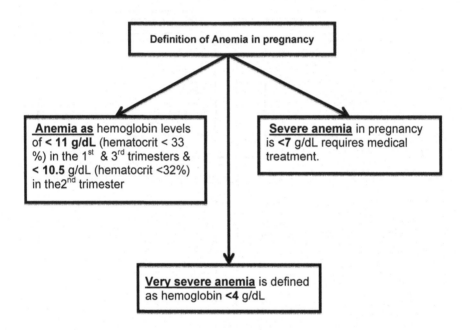

Definition of Anemia in pregnancy

**Anemia as** hemoglobin levels of **< 11 g/dL** (hematocrit < 33 %) in the 1st & 3rd trimesters & **< 10.5** g/dL (hematocrit <32%) in the 2nd trimester

**Severe anemia** in pregnancy is **<7** g/dL requires medical treatment.

**Very severe anemia** is defined as hemoglobin **<4** g/dL

## 5.2    Causes of anemia in pregnancy

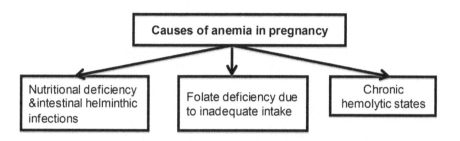

## 5.3    Risk of sever anemia with pregnancy

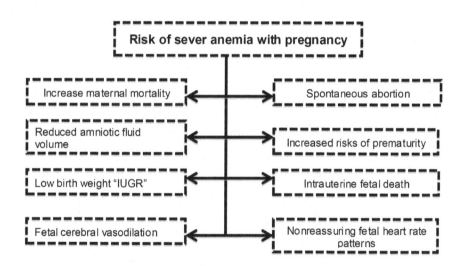

## 5.4   Evaluation of pregnant patient with anemia

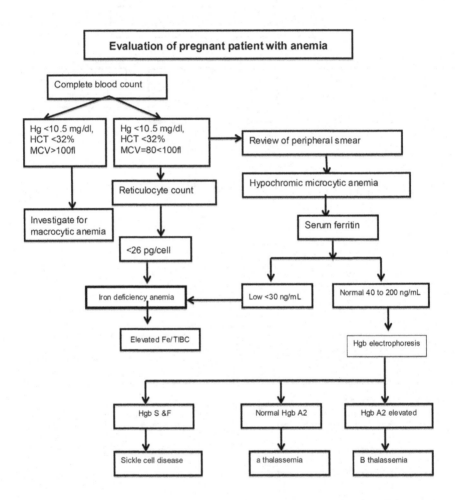

## 5.5   Investigate for macrocytic anemia

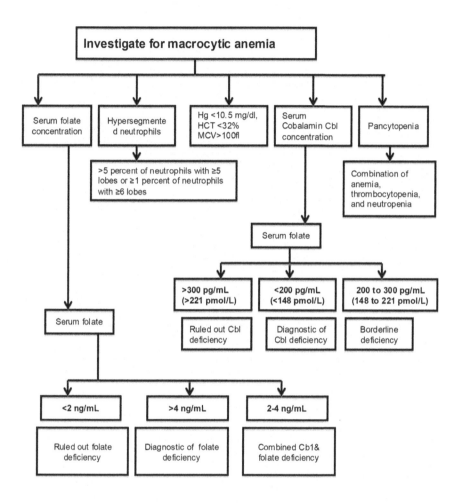

# 5.6    Treatment of anemia in pregnancy

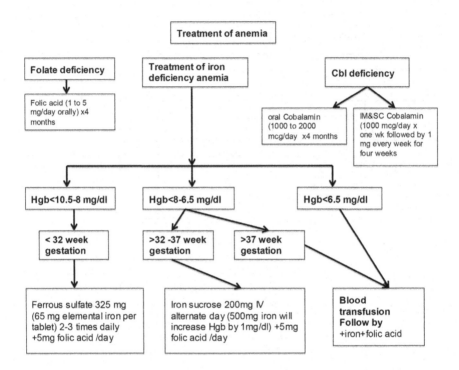

Treatment of anemia

Folate deficiency

Folic acid (1 to 5 mg/day orally) x4 months

Treatment of iron deficiency anemia

Cbl deficiency

oral Cobalamin (1000 to 2000 mcg/day x4 months)

IM&SC Cobalamin (1000 mcg/day x one wk followed by 1 mg every week for four weeks)

Hgb<10.5-8 mg/dl

Hgb<8-6.5 mg/dl

Hgb<6.5 mg/dl

< 32 week gestation

>32 -37 week gestation

>37 week gestation

Ferrous sulfate 325 mg (65 mg elemental iron per tablet) 2-3 times daily +5mg folic acid /day

Iron sucrose 200mg IV alternate day (500mg iron will increase Hgb by 1mg/dl) +5mg folic acid /day

Blood transfusion Follow by +iron+folic acid

# 6   Oligohydramnios

# 6.1   Causes of oligohydramnios

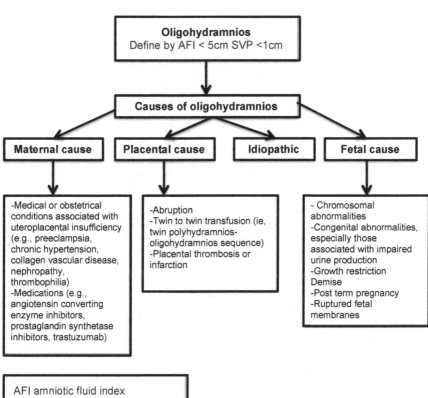

**Oligohydramnios**
Define by AFI < 5cm SVP <1cm

**Causes of oligohydramnios**

**Maternal cause**

**Placental cause**

**Idiopathic**

**Fetal cause**

-Medical or obstetrical conditions associated with uteroplacental insufficiency (e.g., preeclampsia, chronic hypertension, collagen vascular disease, nephropathy, thrombophilia)
-Medications (e.g., angiotensin converting enzyme inhibitors, prostaglandin synthetase inhibitors, trastuzumab)

-Abruption
-Twin to twin transfusion (ie, twin polyhydramnios-oligohydramnios sequence)
-Placental thrombosis or infarction

- Chromosomal abnormalities
-Congenital abnormalities, especially those associated with impaired urine production
-Growth restriction Demise
-Post term pregnancy
-Ruptured fetal membranes

AFI amniotic fluid index
 SVP  single vertical bocket

# 6.2 Management of oligohydramnios

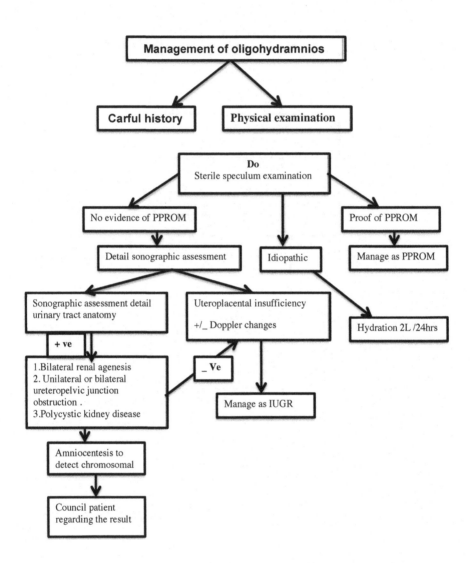

# 7 Polyhydramnios

## 7.1 Causes of oligohydramnios

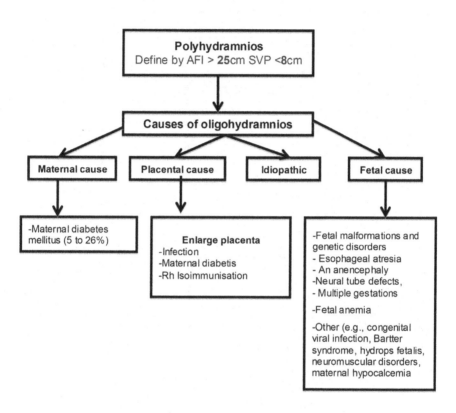

**Polyhydramnios**
Define by AFI > **25**cm SVP <**8**cm

↓

**Causes of oligohydramnios**

**Maternal cause** **Placental cause** **Idiopathic** **Fetal cause**

-Maternal diabetes mellitus (5 to 26%)

**Enlarge placenta**
-Infection
-Maternal diabetis
-Rh Isoimmunisation

-Fetal malformations and genetic disorders
- Esophageal atresia
- An anencephaly
-Neural tube defects,
- Multiple gestations

-Fetal anemia

-Other (e.g., congenital viral infection, Bartter syndrome, hydrops fetalis, neuromuscular disorders, maternal hypocalcemia

# 7.2   Management of polyhydramnios

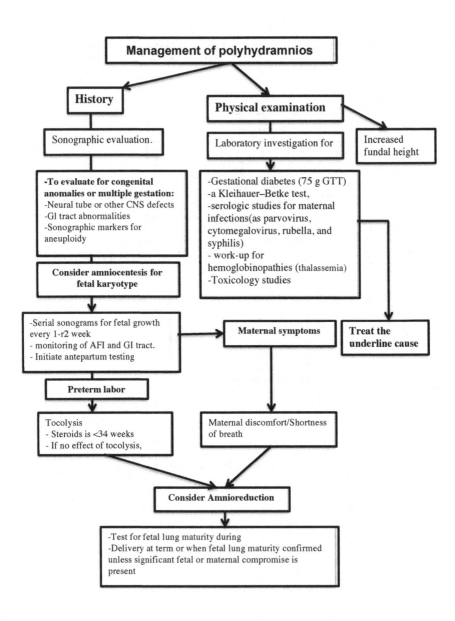

# 8 Intrauterine growth restriction

## 8.1 Management of IUGR

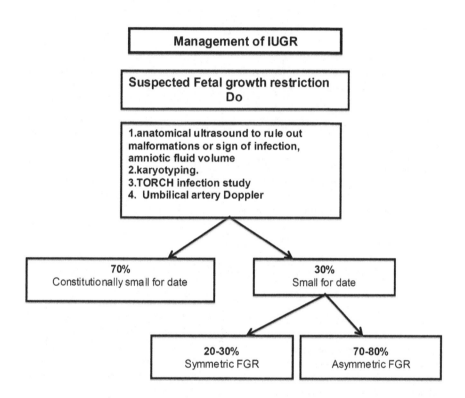

# 8.2  Asymmetrical IUGR

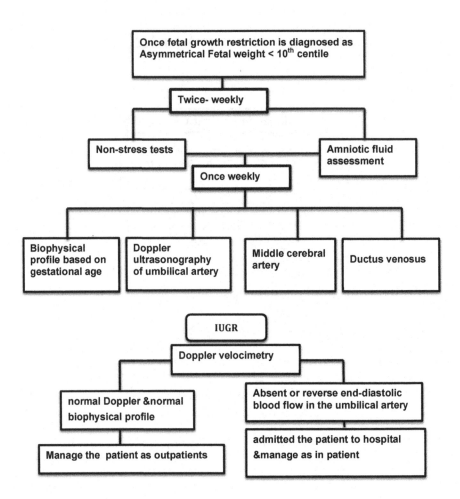

Once fetal growth restriction is diagnosed as Asymmetrical Fetal weight < 10th centile

Twice- weekly

Non-stress tests

Amniotic fluid assessment

Once weekly

Biophysical profile based on gestational age

Doppler ultrasonography of umbilical artery

Middle cerebral artery

Ductus venosus

IUGR

Doppler velocimetry

normal Doppler &normal biophysical profile

Absent or reverse end-diastolic blood flow in the umbilical artery

Manage the patient as outpatients

admitted the patient to hospital &manage as in patient

# 8.3 Management of Asymmetrical IUGR

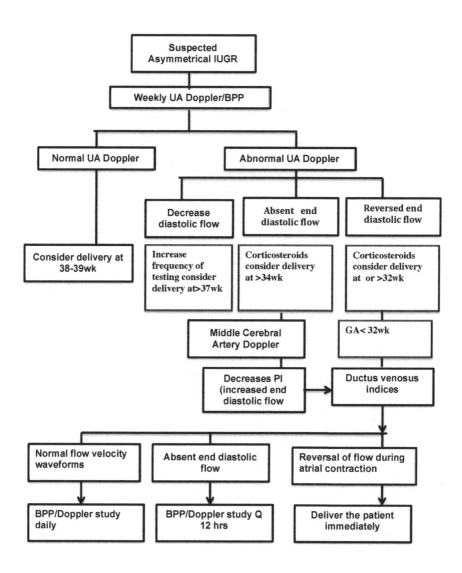

# 9   Urinary tract infections in pregnancy

## 9.1   Type of Urinary tract infections

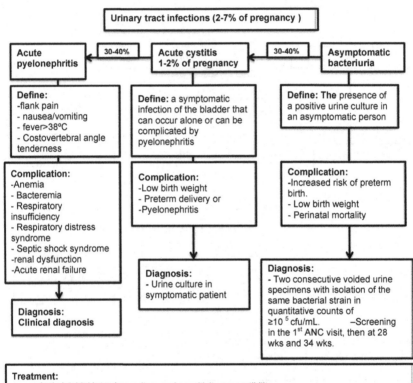

**Urinary tract infections (2-7% of pregnancy )**

**Acute pyelonephritis** ← 30-40% → **Acute cystitis 1-2% of pregnancy** ← 30-40% → **Asymptomatic bacteriuria**

**Define:**
-flank pain
- nausea/vomiting
- fever>38ºC
- Costovertebral angle tenderness

**Define:** a symptomatic infection of the bladder that can occur alone or can be complicated by pyelonephritis

**Define:** The presence of a positive urine culture in an asymptomatic person

**Complication:**
-Anemia
- Bacteremia
- Respiratory insufficiency
- Respiratory distress syndrome
- Septic shock syndrome
-renal dysfunction
-Acute renal failure

**Complication:**
-Low birth weight
- Preterm delivery or
-Pyelonephritis

**Complication:**
-Increased risk of preterm birth.
- Low birth weight
- Perinatal mortality

**Diagnosis:**
- Urine culture in symptomatic patient

**Diagnosis:**
- Two consecutive voided urine specimens with isolation of the same bacterial strain in quantitative counts of ≥10 $^5$ cfu/mL.     —Screening in the 1$^{st}$ ANC visit, then at 28 wks and 34 wks.

**Diagnosis:**
**Clinical diagnosis**

**Treatment:**
- Antimicrobial based on culture and sensitivity susceptibility.
- In acute pyelonephritis 3$^{rd}$ generation cephalosporin is preferred such as cefazolin
- Carbapenems effective in the treatment of  beta lactamase producing strains(meropenem , ertapenem , or doripenem)
-**Acute pyelonephritis** treated for 48hrs by IV antibiotics then shift to oral therapy for 10 days

# 9.2 Management of Urinary tract infections

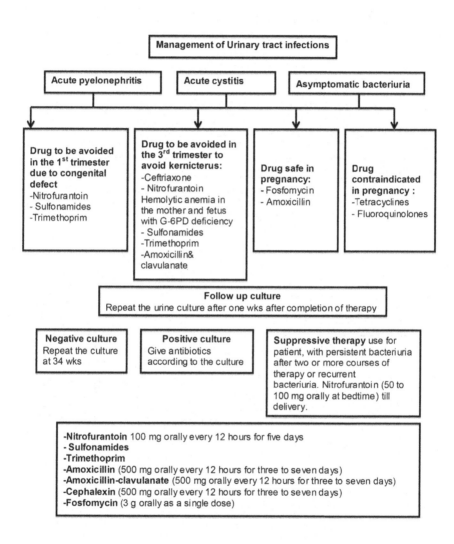

**Management of Urinary tract infections**

**Acute pyelonephritis**  |  **Acute cystitis**  |  **Asymptomatic bacteriuria**

**Drug to be avoided in the 1st trimester due to congenital defect**
-Nitrofurantoin
- Sulfonamides
-Trimethoprim

**Drug to be avoided in the 3rd trimester to avoid kernicterus:**
-Ceftriaxone
- Nitrofurantoin
Hemolytic anemia in the mother and fetus with G-6PD deficiency
- Sulfonamides
-Trimethoprim
-Amoxicillin& clavulanate

**Drug safe in pregnancy:**
- Fosfomycin
- Amoxicillin

**Drug contraindicated in pregnancy :**
-Tetracyclines
- Fluoroquinolones

**Follow up culture**
Repeat the urine culture after one wks after completion of therapy

**Negative culture**
Repeat the culture at 34 wks

**Positive culture**
Give antibiotics according to the culture

**Suppressive therapy** use for patient, with persistent bacteriuria after two or more courses of therapy or recurrent bacteriuria. Nitrofurantoin (50 to 100 mg orally at bedtime) till delivery.

-**Nitrofurantoin** 100 mg orally every 12 hours for five days
- **Sulfonamides**
-**Trimethoprim**
-**Amoxicillin** (500 mg orally every 12 hours for three to seven days)
-**Amoxicillin-clavulanate** (500 mg orally every 12 hours for three to seven days)
-**Cephalexin** (500 mg orally every 12 hours for three to seven days)
-**Fosfomycin** (3 g orally as a single dose)

# 10    Intrahepatic cholestasis of pregnancy

## 10.1    Management of Intrahepatic cholestasis of pregnancy

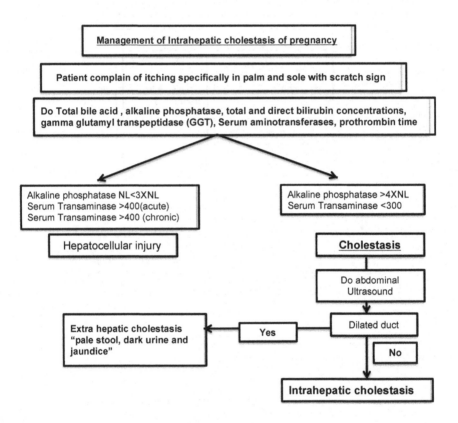

## 10.2   Management of Intrahepatic cholestasis of pregnancy2

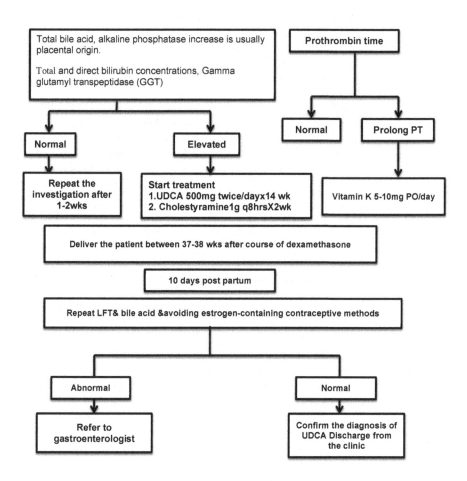

# 11   Varicella-zoster virus in pregnancy

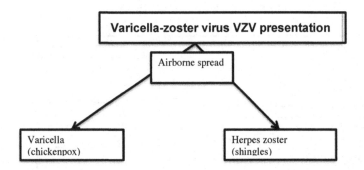

Varicella-zoster virus VZV presentation

Airborne spread

Varicella
(chickenpox)

Herpes zoster
(shingles)

Incubation period is 14–16 days
-contagious from 1–2 days before to
after onset of the rash
-patient may develop fever, malaise,
and a pruritic maculopapular rash then
rapidly form vesicles then crust

Incubation period is 14–16 days
-Painful skin lesions over the areas of
distribution of one or more sensory nerve
roots                                      -The
eruption is  unilateral but  sometimes
cross the midline.

# 11.1   VZV complication

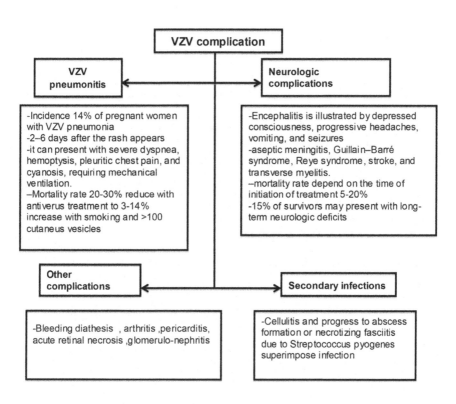

**VZV complication**

**VZV pneumonitis**

-Incidence 14% of pregnant women with VZV pneumonia
-2–6 days after the rash appears
-it can present with severe dyspnea, hemoptysis, pleuritic chest pain, and cyanosis, requiring mechanical ventilation.
–Mortality rate 20-30% reduce with antiverus treatment to 3-14% increase with smoking and >100 cutaneus vesicles

**Neurologic complications**

-Encephalitis is illustrated by depressed consciousness, progressive headaches, vomiting, and seizures
-aseptic meningitis, Guillain–Barré syndrome, Reye syndrome, stroke, and transverse myelitis.
–mortality rate depend on the time of initiation of treatment 5-20%
-15% of survivors may present with long-term neurologic deficits

**Other complications**

-Bleeding diathesis , arthritis ,pericarditis, acute retinal necrosis ,glomerulo-nephritis

**Secondary infections**

-Cellulitis and progress to abscess formation or necrotizing fasciitis due to Streptococcus pyogenes superimpose infection

# 11.2   VZV diagnosis

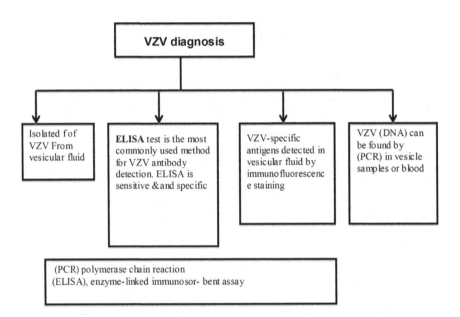

**VZV diagnosis**

Isolated f of VZV From vesicular fluid

**ELISA** test is the most commonly used method for VZV antibody detection. ELISA is sensitive &and specific

VZV-specific antigens detected in vesicular fluid by immunofluorescence staining

VZV (DNA) can be found by (PCR) in vesicle samples or blood

(PCR) polymerase chain reaction
(ELISA), enzyme-linked immunosor- bent assay

# 11.3   VZV Treatment

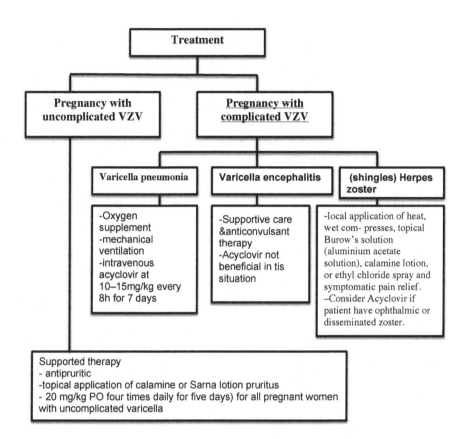

**Treatment**

**Pregnancy with uncomplicated VZV**

**Pregnancy with complicated VZV**

**Varicella pneumonia**

-Oxygen supplement
-mechanical ventilation
-intravenous acyclovir at 10–15mg/kg every 8h for 7 days

**Varicella encephalitis**

-Supportive care &anticonvulsant therapy
-Acyclovir not beneficial in tis situation

**(shingles) Herpes zoster**

-local application of heat, wet com- presses, topical Burow's solution (aluminium acetate solution), calamine lotion, or ethyl chloride spray and symptomatic pain relief.
–Consider Acyclovir if patient have ophthalmic or disseminated zoster.

Supported therapy
- antipruritic
-topical application of calamine or Sarna lotion pruritus
- 20 mg/kg PO four times daily for five days) for all pregnant women with uncomplicated varicella

# 11.4   Management of VZV Exposure during pregnancy

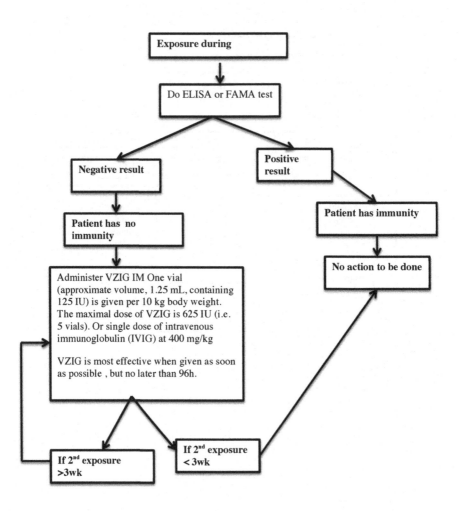

Exposure during

↓

Do ELISA or FAMA test

Negative result

Positive result

Patient has no immunity

Patient has immunity

Administer VZIG IM One vial (approximate volume, 1.25 mL, containing 125 IU) is given per 10 kg body weight. The maximal dose of VZIG is 625 IU (i.e. 5 vials). Or single dose of intravenous immunoglobulin (IVIG) at 400 mg/kg

VZIG is most effective when given as soon as possible , but no later than 96h.

No action to be done

If 2$^{nd}$ exposure >3wk

If 2$^{nd}$ exposure < 3wk

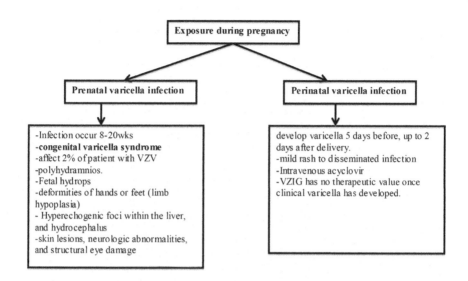

# 12   Toxoplasmosis and pregnancy

## 12.1   Toxoplasma infection during pregnancy

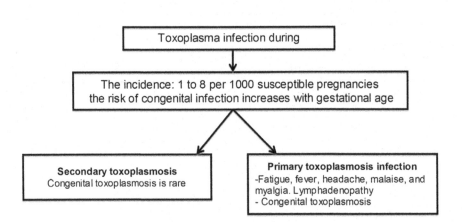

# 12.2   Toxoplasma infection diagnosis

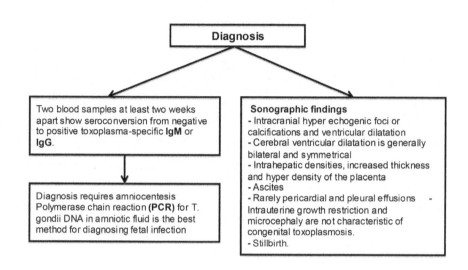

**Diagnosis**

Two blood samples at least two weeks apart show seroconversion from negative to positive toxoplasma-specific **IgM** or **IgG**.

Diagnosis requires amniocentesis Polymerase chain reaction **(PCR)** for T. gondii DNA in amniotic fluid is the best method for diagnosing fetal infection

**Sonographic findings**
- Intracranial hyper echogenic foci or calcifications and ventricular dilatation
- Cerebral ventricular dilatation is generally bilateral and symmetrical
- Intrahepatic densities, increased thickness and hyper density of the placenta
- Ascites
- Rarely pericardial and pleural effusions    - Intrauterine growth restriction and microcephaly are not characteristic of congenital toxoplasmosis.
- Stillbirth.

# 12.3   Tratment of Toxoplasma infection during pregnancy

---

**Treatment**

Infected during pregnancy are generally treated immediately with **spiramycin** (1 g orally every eight hours without food)
**Pyrimethamine** is a folic acid antagonist which can cause dose-related bone marrow suppression with resultant anemia, leukopenia, and thrombocytopenia
**Sulfadiazine**, can cause bone marrow suppression and reversible acute renal failure

---

**Treatment**

-Early treatment patients don't reduced the risk of intracranial lesions detected after birth, or of retinochoroiditis detected during infancy or mother-to-child transmission of infection -There is clear evidence that treatment reduce serious neurological sequelae or postnatal death in children with congenital toxoplasmosis

---

# 13   Gonorrheal infection in pregnancy

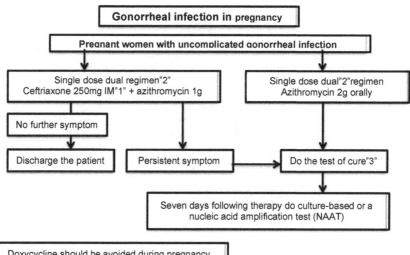

Gonorrheal infection in pregnancy

Pregnant women with uncomplicated gonorrheal infection

Single dose dual regimen"2"
Ceftriaxone 250mg IM"1" + azithromycin 1g

Single dose dual"2"regimen
Azithromycin 2g orally

No further symptom

Discharge the patient

Persistent symptom

Do the test of cure"3"

Seven days following therapy do culture-based or a nucleic acid amplification test (NAAT)

Doxycycline should be avoided during pregnancy

All pregnant women with pelvic inflammatory disease should be hospitalized and given parenteral antibiotics, due to the potential complications of infection resulting in adverse pregnancy outcomes.

## 14    Hepatitis B during pregnancy

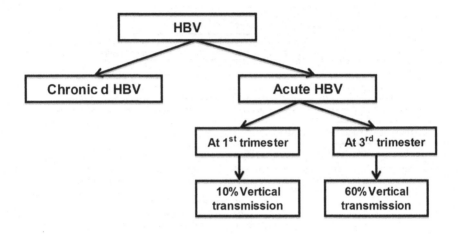

# 14.1    Management of acute HBV

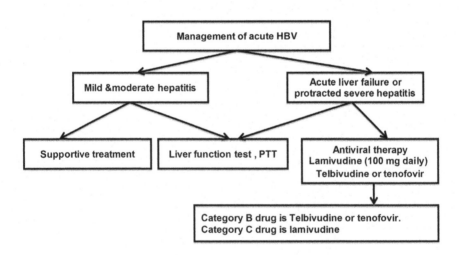

# 14.2   Chronic HBV

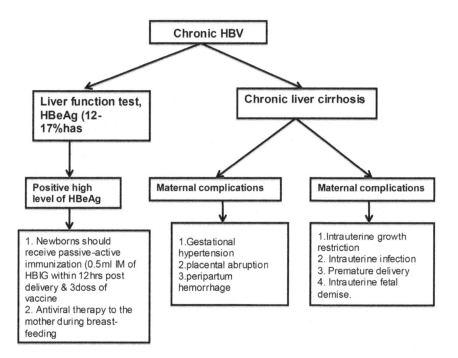

Chronic HBV

Liver function test, HBeAg (12-17%has

Chronic liver cirrhosis

Positive high level of HBeAg

1. Newborns should receive passive-active immunization (0.5ml IM of HBIG within 12hrs post delivery & 3doss of vaccine
2. Antiviral therapy to the mother during breast-feeding

Maternal complications

1.Gestational hypertension
2.placental abruption
3.peripartum hemorrhage

Maternal complications

1.Intrauterine growth restriction
2. Intrauterine infection
3. Premature delivery
4. Intrauterine fetal demise.

## 14.3  Breast-feeding in patient with HBV

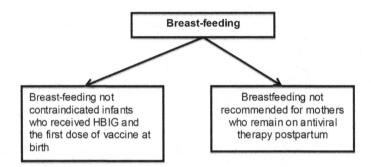

Dose of HBIG (0.06 ml/kg or 5.0 ml for adults) after accidental exposure to blood contaminated with hepatitis B

# 15 Cytomegalovirus infection in pregnancy

# 15.1 Cytomegalovirus infection (CMV)

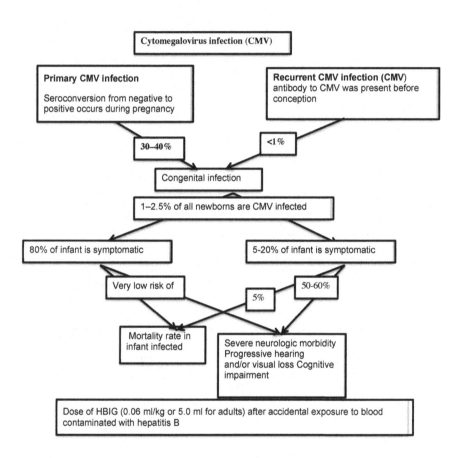

# 15.2   Maternal CMV infection

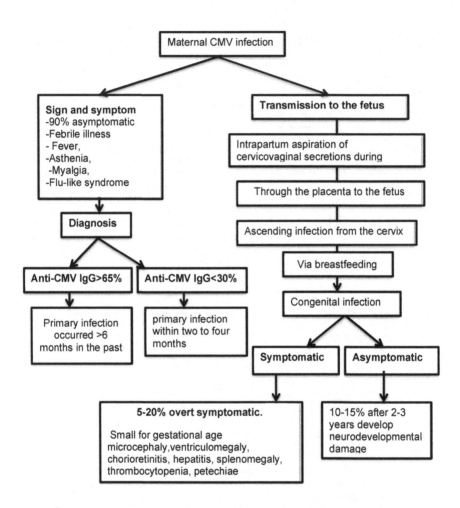

# 15.3 Prenatal diagnosis

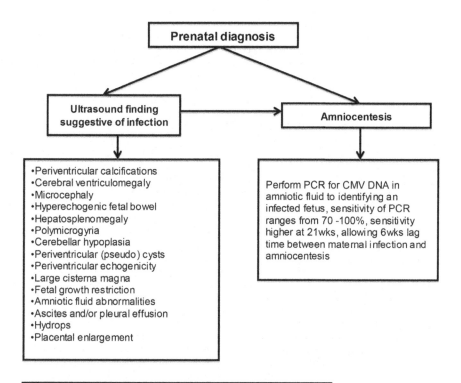

```
                    ┌──────────────────────────┐
                    │    Prenatal diagnosis    │
                    └──────────────────────────┘
```

**Ultrasound finding suggestive of infection**

**Amniocentesis**

- Periventricular calcifications
- Cerebral ventriculomegaly
- Microcephaly
- Hyperechogenic fetal bowel
- Hepatosplenomegaly
- Polymicrogyria
- Cerebellar hypoplasia
- Periventricular (pseudo) cysts
- Periventricular echogenicity
- Large cisterna magna
- Fetal growth restriction
- Amniotic fluid abnormalities
- Ascites and/or pleural effusion
- Hydrops
- Placental enlargement

Perform PCR for CMV DNA in amniotic fluid to identifying an infected fetus, sensitivity of PCR ranges from 70 -100%, sensitivity higher at 21wks, allowing 6wks lag time between maternal infection and amniocentesis

During pregnancy, there is no effective treatment for prevention of fetal disease or reduction in risk of sequelae of CMV.

## 16.1   Genital herpes simplex virus (HSV) infection

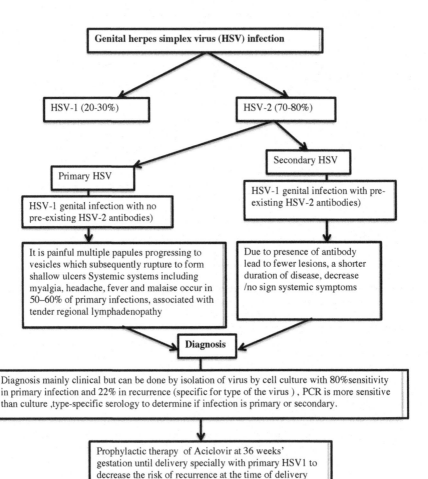

Genital herpes simplex virus (HSV) infection

HSV-1 (20-30%)

HSV-2 (70-80%)

Primary HSV

Secondary HSV

HSV-1 genital infection with no pre-existing HSV-2 antibodies)

HSV-1 genital infection with pre-existing HSV-2 antibodies)

It is painful multiple papules progressing to vesicles which subsequently rupture to form shallow ulcers Systemic systems including myalgia, headache, fever and malaise occur in 50–60% of primary infections, associated with tender regional lymphadenopathy

Due to presence of antibody lead to fewer lesions, a shorter duration of disease, decrease /no sign systemic symptoms

Diagnosis

Diagnosis mainly clinical but can be done by isolation of virus by cell culture with 80%sensitivity in primary infection and 22% in recurrence (specific for type of the virus ) , PCR is more sensitive than culture ,type-specific serology to determine if infection is primary or secondary.

Prophylactic therapy of Aciclovir at 36 weeks' gestation until delivery specially with primary HSV1 to decrease the risk of recurrence at the time of delivery

# 16.2   Genital Herpes during Labour or <34 weeks gestation

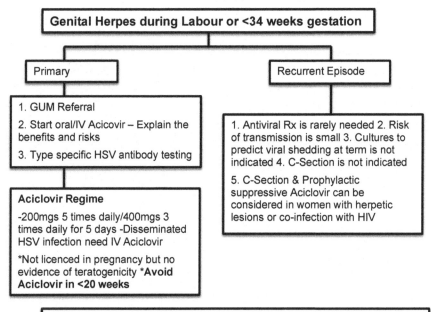

**Genital Herpes during Labour or <34 weeks gestation**

**Primary**

1. GUM Referral
2. Start oral/IV Acicovir – Explain the benefits and risks
3. Type specific HSV antibody testing

**Aciclovir Regime**

-200mgs 5 times daily/400mgs 3 times daily for 5 days -Disseminated HSV infection need IV Aciclovir

*Not licenced in pregnancy but no evidence of teratogenicity **Avoid Aciclovir in <20 weeks**

**Recurrent Episode**

1. Antiviral Rx is rarely needed 2. Risk of transmission is small 3. Cultures to predict viral shedding at term is not indicated 4. C-Section is not indicated

5. C-Section & Prophylactic suppressive Aciclovir can be considered in women with herpetic lesions or co-infection with HIV

**Abbreviations**

GUM- Genito Urinary Medicine ARM- Artificial Rupture of Membranes HSV- Herpes Simplex Virus FSE- Fetal Scalp Electrode HIV- Human Immunodeficiency Virus FBS- Fetal Blood Sampling

# 16.3   Genital Herpes at >34 weeks

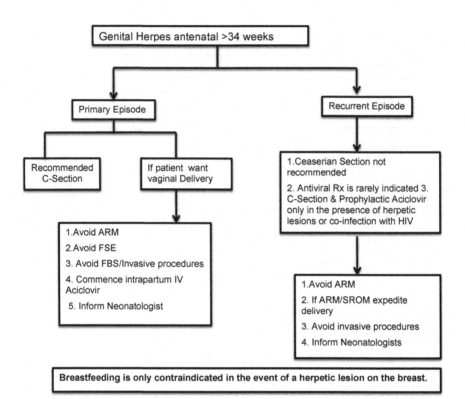

Genital Herpes antenatal >34 weeks

Primary Episode

Recurrent Episode

Recommended C-Section

If patient want vaginal Delivery

1.Ceaserian Section not recommended

2. Antiviral Rx is rarely indicated 3. C-Section & Prophylactic Aciclovir only in the presence of herpetic lesions or co-infection with HIV

1.Avoid ARM

2.Avoid FSE

3. Avoid FBS/Invasive procedures

4. Commence intrapartum IV Aciclovir

 5. Inform Neonatologist

1.Avoid ARM

2. If ARM/SROM expedite delivery

3. Avoid invasive procedures

4. Inform Neonatologists

**Breastfeeding is only contraindicated in the event of a herpetic lesion on the breast.**

# 17 Parvovirus B19 infection

## 17.1 Parvovirus B19 infection

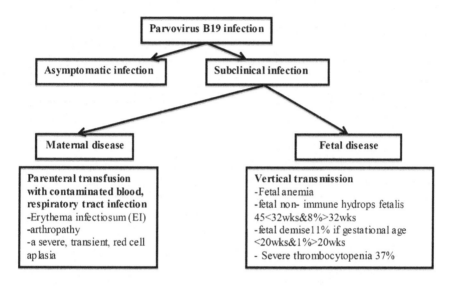

# 17.2   Parvovirus B19 infection diagnosia

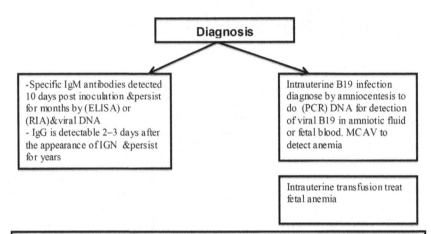

Diagnosis

-Specific IgM antibodies detected 10 days post inoculation &persist for months by (ELISA) or (RIA)&viral DNA
- IgG is detectable 2–3 days after the appearance of IGN &persist for years

Intrauterine B19 infection diagnose by amniocentesis to do (PCR) DNA for detection of viral B19 in amniotic fluid or fetal blood. MCAV to detect anemia

Intrauterine transfusion treat fetal anemia

Enzyme-linked immune absorbent assay (ELISA) or radioimmunoassay (RIA), and viral DNA, polymerase chain reaction (PCR),MCAV middle cerebral artery Doppler velocimetry

# 18   Syphilis in pregnancy

# 18.1   Stages of Syphilis during pregnancy

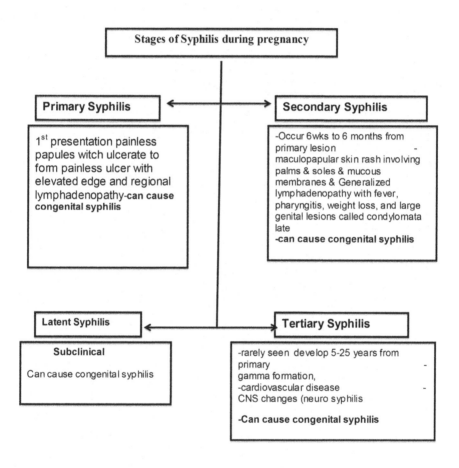

**Stages of Syphilis during pregnancy**

**Primary Syphilis**

1<sup>st</sup> presentation painless papules witch ulcerate to form painless ulcer with elevated edge and regional lymphadenopathy-**can cause congenital syphilis**

**Secondary Syphilis**

-Occur 6wks to 6 months from primary lesion                -maculopapular skin rash involving palms & soles & mucous membranes & Generalized lymphadenopathy with fever, pharyngitis, weight loss, and large genital lesions called condylomata late
**-can cause congenital syphilis**

**Latent Syphilis**

**Subclinical**

Can cause congenital syphilis

**Tertiary Syphilis**

-rarely seen develop 5-25 years from primary                -gamma formation,
-cardiovascular disease            -CNS changes (neuro syphilis

**-Can cause congenital syphilis**

# 18.2   Syphilis complicating pregnancy

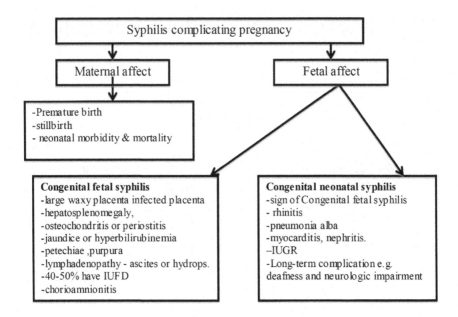

**Syphilis complicating pregnancy**

**Maternal affect**

- Premature birth
- stillbirth
- neonatal morbidity & mortality

**Fetal affect**

**Congenital fetal syphilis**
- large waxy placenta infected placenta
- hepatosplenomegaly,
- osteochondritis or periostitis
- jaundice or hyperbilirubinemia
- petechiae ,purpura
- lymphadenopathy - ascites or hydrops.
- 40-50% have IUFD
- chorioamnionitis

**Congenital neonatal syphilis**
- sign of Congenital fetal syphilis
- rhinitis
- pneumonia alba
- myocarditis, nephritis.
- –IUGR
- Long-term complication e.g.
deafness and neurologic impairment

# 18.3   Syphilis Diagnosis

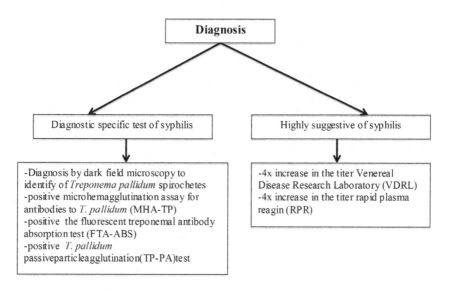

Diagnosis

Diagnostic specific test of syphilis

-Diagnosis by dark field microscopy to
identify of *Treponema pallidum* spirochetes
-positive microhemagglutination assay for
antibodies to *T. pallidum* (MHA-TP)
-positive the fluorescent treponemal antibody
absorption test (FTA-ABS)
-positive *T. pallidum*
passiveparticleagglutination(TP-PA)test

Highly suggestive of syphilis

-4x increase in the titer Venereal
Disease Research Laboratory (VDRL)
-4x increase in the titer rapid plasma
reagin (RPR)

# 18.4   Management of syphilis in pregnancy

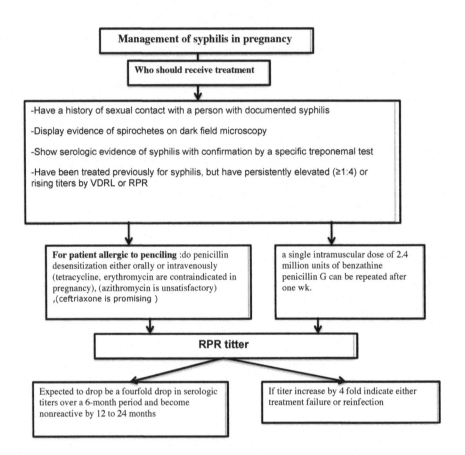

**Management of syphilis in pregnancy**

**Who should receive treatment**

-Have a history of sexual contact with a person with documented syphilis

-Display evidence of spirochetes on dark field microscopy

-Show serologic evidence of syphilis with confirmation by a specific treponemal test

-Have been treated previously for syphilis, but have persistently elevated (≥1:4) or rising titers by VDRL or RPR

**For patient allergic to penciling** :do penicillin desensitization either orally or intravenously (tetracycline, erythromycin are contraindicated in pregnancy), (azithromycin is unsatisfactory) ,(ceftriaxone is promising )

a single intramuscular dose of 2.4 million units of benzathine penicillin G can be repeated after one wk.

**RPR titter**

Expected to drop be a fourfold drop in serologic titers over a 6-month period and become nonreactive by 12 to 24 months

If titer increase by 4 fold indicate either treatment failure or reinfection

# 19  Sickle cell disease with pregnancy

## 19.1  Prepregnancy evaluation of sickle cell disease

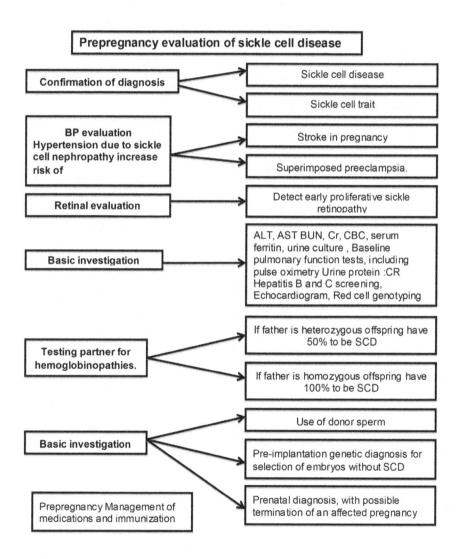

# 19.2 Prepregnancy Management of medications & immunization in sickle cell disease patient

| Prepregnancy Management of medications & immunization | |
|---|---|
| Immunization | Give the vaccine for polyvalent pneumococcal; Haemophilus influenza type B, and meningococcal vaccines avoid pregnancy for four weeks after administration of a live vaccine. |
| Folic acid | Recommended dose 5mg /day |
| Iron chelators | Discontinue iron chelation therapy once conceive |
| Hydroxyurea | Discontinue hydroxyurea three months before conception |
| ACE inhibitors and ARBs | Discontinue this medication because it is teratogenicity |
| Prophylactic penicillin | penicillin therapy may be continued during pregnancy |
| Analgesia | NSAIDs avoided after 30 wks because of the risk of premature closure of ductus arteriosus |

# 19.3   Risk of sickle cell disease on pregnancy

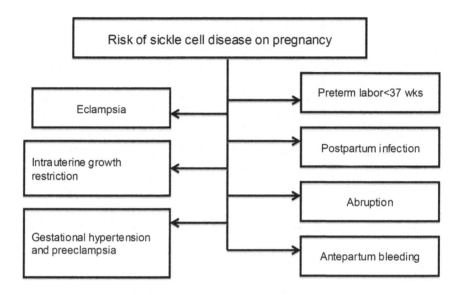

Risk of sickle cell disease on pregnancy

Eclampsia

Preterm labor<37 wks

Intrauterine growth restriction

Postpartum infection

Abruption

Gestational hypertension and preeclampsia

Antepartum bleeding

# 19.4   Prenatal care of sickle cell disease "HbSS, HbSC, HbS/beta-thal

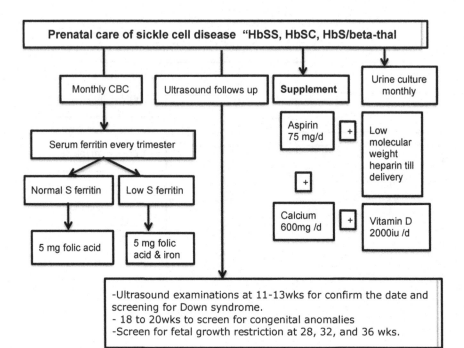

Prenatal care of sickle cell disease  "HbSS, HbSC, HbS/beta-thal

Monthly CBC

Ultrasound follows up

**Supplement**

Urine culture monthly

Serum ferritin every trimester

Normal S ferritin

Low S ferritin

5 mg folic acid

5 mg folic acid & iron

Aspirin 75 mg/d

+

Low molecular weight heparin till delivery

+

Calcium 600mg /d

+

Vitamin D 2000iu /d

-Ultrasound examinations at 11-13wks for confirm the date and screening for Down syndrome.
- 18 to 20wks to screen for congenital anomalies
-Screen for fetal growth restriction at 28, 32, and 36 wks.

# 19.5 Management of complication

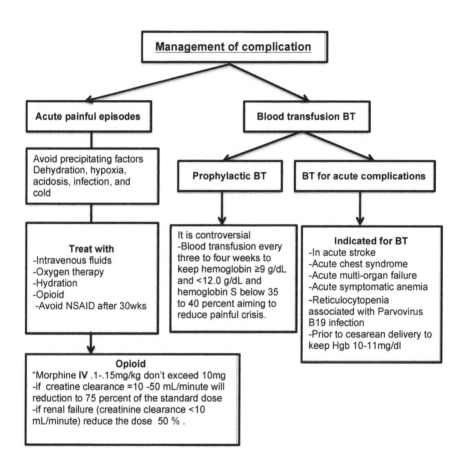

**Management of complication**

**Acute painful episodes**

**Blood transfusion BT**

**Prophylactic BT**

**BT for acute complications**

Avoid precipitating factors Dehydration, hypoxia, acidosis, infection, and cold

**Treat with**
-Intravenous fluids
-Oxygen therapy
-Hydration
-Opioid
-Avoid NSAID after 30wks

It is controversial
-Blood transfusion every three to four weeks to keep hemoglobin ≥9 g/dL and <12.0 g/dL and hemoglobin S below 35 to 40 percent aiming to reduce painful crisis.

**Indicated for BT**
-In acute stroke
-Acute chest syndrome
-Acute multi-organ failure
-Acute symptomatic anemia
-Reticulocytopenia associated with Parvovirus B19 infection
-Prior to cesarean delivery to keep Hgb 10-11mg/dl

**Opioid**
"Morphine IV .1-.15mg/kg don't exceed 10mg
-if creatine clearance =10 -50 mL/minute will reduction to 75 percent of the standard dose
-if renal failure (creatinine clearance <10 mL/minute) reduce the dose 50 % .

# 20 Hypothyroidism

## 20.1 Hypothyroidism in preconception

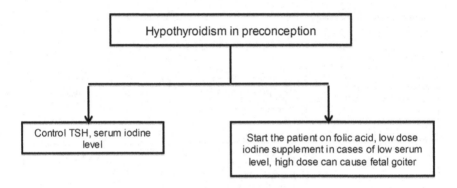

Hypothyroidism in preconception

Control TSH, serum iodine level

Start the patient on folic acid, low dose iodine supplement in cases of low serum level, high dose can cause fetal goiter

# 20.2　Thyroid disease in pregnancy

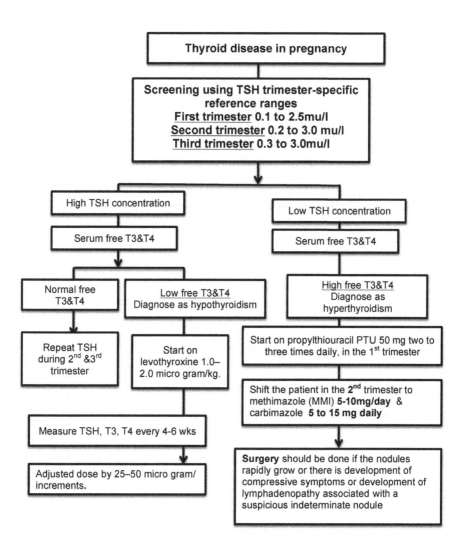

Thyroid disease in pregnancy

Screening using TSH trimester-specific reference ranges
**First trimester** 0.1 to 2.5mu/l
**Second trimester** 0.2 to 3.0 mu/l
**Third trimester** 0.3 to 3.0mu/l

High TSH concentration

Serum free T3&T4

Normal free T3&T4

Low free T3&T4
Diagnose as hypothyroidism

Repeat TSH during 2nd &3rd trimester

Start on levothyroxine 1.0–2.0 micro gram/kg.

Measure TSH, T3, T4 every 4-6 wks

Adjusted dose by 25–50 micro gram/ increments.

Low TSH concentration

Serum free T3&T4

High free T3&T4
Diagnose as hyperthyroidism

Start on propylthiouracil PTU 50 mg two to three times daily, in the 1st trimester

Shift the patient in the 2nd trimester to methimazole (MMI) **5-10mg/day** & carbimazole **5 to 15 mg daily**

**Surgery** should be done if the nodules rapidly grow or there is development of compressive symptoms or development of lymphadenopathy associated with a suspicious indeterminate nodule

# 21   Diabetes

## 21.1   Gestational diabetes

| Gestational diabetes |
| :---: |

| Preconception visit |
| :---: |

1.A family history of diabetes, especially in first degree relatives

2.Prepregnancy weight ≥110 percent of ideal body weight or body mass index >30 kg/m 2 or excessive gestational weight gain

3.Age >25 years

4.Previous delivery of a baby >9 pounds [4.1 kg]

5.Personal history of impaired glucose tolerance

6.Member of an ethnic group with higher than the background rate of type 2 diabetes (eg, Hispanic-American, African-American, Native American, South or East Asian, Pacific Islander).

7.Previous unexplained perinatal loss or birth of a malformed infant

8.Maternal birthweight >9 pounds [4.1 kg] or <6 pounds [2.7 kg]

9.Glycosuria at the first prenatal visit

10.Polycystic ovary syndrome

11.Current use of glucocorticoids

12.Essential hypertension or pregnancy-related hypertension

13.Metabolic syndrome

If the patient has one or more risk factor screen for gestational diabetis A1C

# 21.2   screen for gestational diabetis

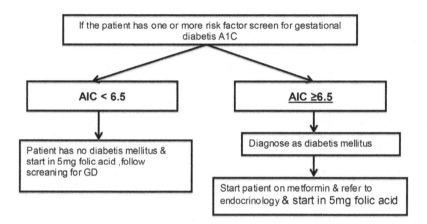

If the patient has one or more risk factor screen for gestational diabetis A1C

**AIC < 6.5**

**AIC ≥6.5**

Patient has no diabetis mellitus & start in 5mg folic acid ,follow screaning for GD

Diagnose as diabetis mellitus

Start patient on metformin & refer to endocrinology & start in 5mg folic acid

---

**Normal value for BSP** FBS<92 mg/dL (5.1 mmol/L) 2hrs postprandial 2-h <140 mg/dl (7.7 mmol)

---

**75g GTT** normal value ( one abnormal value will consider the patient gestational diabetis
**Fasting plasma glucose** ≥92 mg/dL [5.1 mmol/L], **one hour** ≥180 mg/dL (10.0 mmol/L) **two hour** ≥153 mg/dL (8.5 mmol/L)

# 21.3 Follow up of gestational diabetis

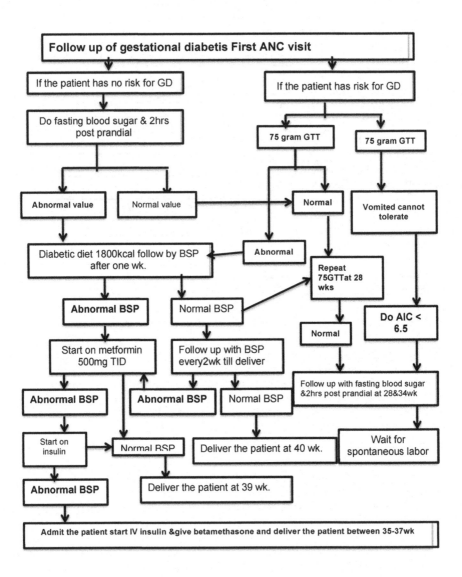

# 22 Preconception type 1&type 2 diabetes mellitus

## 22.1 Preconception management of type 1&type 2 diabetes mellitus

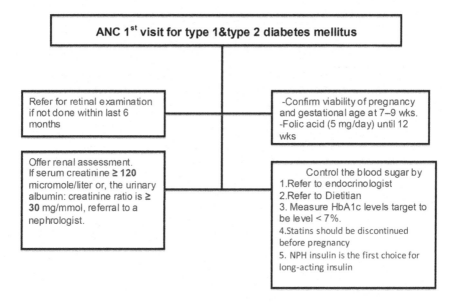

ANC 1st visit for type 1&type 2 diabetes mellitus

Refer for retinal examination if not done within last 6 months

-Confirm viability of pregnancy and gestational age at 7–9 wks.
-Folic acid (5 mg/day) until 12 wks

Offer renal assessment. If serum creatinine ≥ **120** micromole/liter or, the urinary albumin: creatinine ratio is ≥ **30** mg/mmol, referral to a nephrologist.

Control the blood sugar by
1.Refer to endocrinologist
2.Refer to Dietitian
3. Measure HbA1c levels target to be level < 7%.
4.Statins should be discontinued before pregnancy
5. NPH insulin is the first choice for long-acting insulin

## 22.2   Preconception management of type 1&type 2 diabetes mellitus

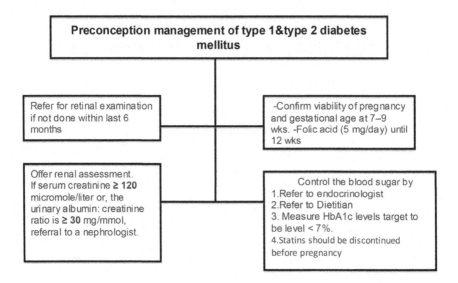

## 22.3   ANC follow up for type 1&type 2 diabetes mellitus

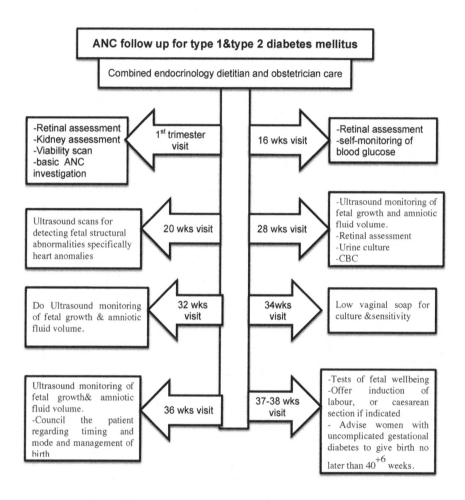

ANC follow up for type 1&type 2 diabetes mellitus

Combined endocrinology dietitian and obstetrician care

-Retinal assessment
-Kidney assessment
-Viability scan
-basic ANC investigation

1st trimester visit

16 wks visit

-Retinal assessment
-self-monitoring of blood glucose

Ultrasound scans for detecting fetal structural abnormalities specifically heart anomalies

20 wks visit

28 wks visit

-Ultrasound monitoring of fetal growth and amniotic fluid volume.
-Retinal assessment
-Urine culture
-CBC

Do Ultrasound monitoring of fetal growth & amniotic fluid volume.

32 wks visit

34wks visit

Low vaginal soap for culture &sensitivity

Ultrasound monitoring of fetal growth& amniotic fluid volume.
-Council the patient regarding timing and mode and management of birth

36 wks visit

37-38 wks visit

-Tests of fetal wellbeing
-Offer induction of labour, or caesarean section if indicated
- Advise women with uncomplicated gestational diabetes to give birth no later than $40^{+6}$ weeks.

# 22.4   Intrapartum care for patient with diabetis mellitus

| Intrapartum care |
|---|

**Counseling regarding the time of delivery**
→
1. uncomplicated gestational diabetes to deliver at 40 wks, 2.patient with insulin to be induce between 37 -38 wks
3. poor control diabetic patient with history of recurrent hypoglycemic attach 35 wks will be appropriate time

**Counseling regarding antenatal steroids**
→
Antenatal steroids for fetal lung maturation is not contraindicated for patient with type 1&2 diabetis mellitus ,but additional insulin should be consider in such patient

**Counseling regarding fetal macrosomia complication**
→
Antenatal steroids for fetal lung maturation is not contraindicated for patient with type 1&2 diabetis mellitus ,but additional insulin should be consider in such patient

**Counseling regarding vaginal delivery after ceaserian section**
→
Diabetes should not in itself be considered a contraindication to attempting vaginal birth after a previous caesarean section

# 22.5 Post natal care with diabetis mellitus type1&2

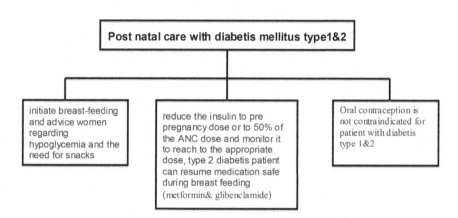

Post natal care with diabetis mellitus type1&2

initiate breast-feeding and advice women regarding hypoglycemia and the need for snacks

reduce the insulin to pre pregnancy dose or to 50% of the ANC dose and monitor it to reach to the appropriate dose, type 2 diabetis patient can resume medication safe during breast feeding (metformin& glibenclamide)

Oral contraception is not contraindicated for patient with diabetis type 1&2

# 23   Hypertension in pregnancy

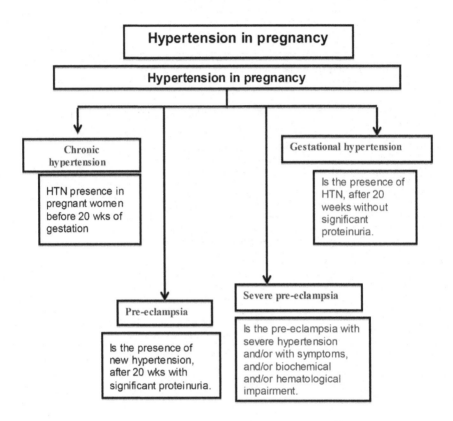

**Hypertension in pregnancy**

Hypertension in pregnancy

**Chronic hypertension**

HTN presence in pregnant women before 20 wks of gestation

**Gestational hypertension**

Is the presence of HTN, after 20 weeks without significant proteinuria.

**Pre-eclampsia**

Is the presence of new hypertension, after 20 wks with significant proteinuria.

**Severe pre-eclampsia**

Is the pre-eclampsia with severe hypertension and/or with symptoms, and/or biochemical and/or hematological impairment.

## 23.1   Risk factors for pre-eclampsia

The risk factors for pre-eclampsia

1.Hypertensive disease during a previous pregnancy

2.Chronic kidney disease

3.Autoimmune disease such as systemic lupus erythematosus or antiphospholipid syndrome

4.Type 1 or type 2 diabetes

5.Chronic hypertension.

**Advise women at high risk of pre-eclampsia to take 81 mg of aspirin**

**-Women with chronic HTN advice to stop angiotensin-converting enzyme (ACE) because of risk of congenital anomalies**

## 23.2   HTN disease in pregnancy

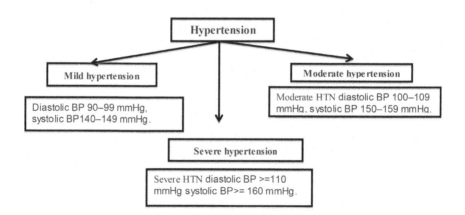

# 23.3   Chronic hypertension in pregnancy

**<u>Management of chronic HTN during pregnancy</u>**

**<u>ANC follow up</u>**

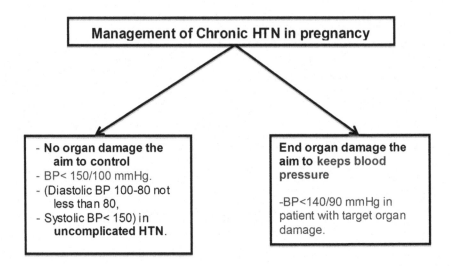

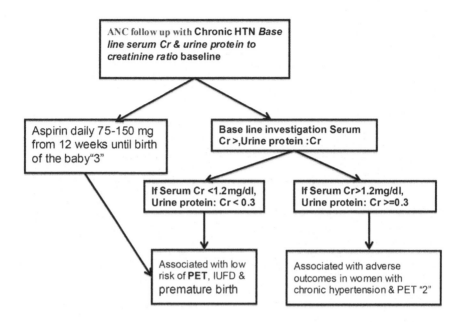

Referral to a specialist in hypertensive disorders in-patient with secondary chronic   HTN

# 23.4 Antihypertensive drug during pregnancy

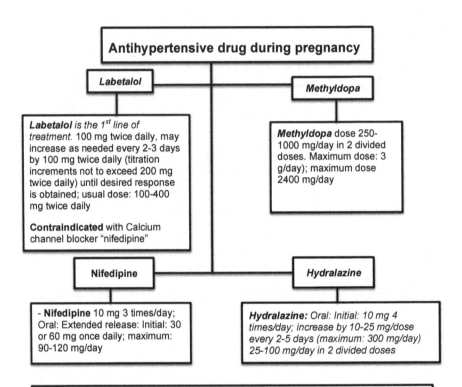

**Antihypertensive drug during pregnancy**

**Labetalol**

**Labetalol** is the 1$^{st}$ line of treatment. 100 mg twice daily, may increase as needed every 2-3 days by 100 mg twice daily (titration increments not to exceed 200 mg twice daily) until desired response is obtained; usual dose: 100-400 mg twice daily

**Contraindicated** with Calcium channel blocker "nifedipine"

**Methyldopa**

**Methyldopa** dose 250-1000 mg/day in 2 divided doses. Maximum dose: 3 g/day); maximum dose 2400 mg/day

**Nifedipine**

- **Nifedipine** 10 mg 3 times/day; Oral: Extended release: Initial: 30 or 60 mg once daily; maximum: 90-120 mg/day

**Hydralazine**

**Hydralazine:** Oral: Initial: 10 mg 4 times/day; increase by 10-25 mg/dose every 2-5 days (maximum: 300 mg/day) 25-100 mg/day in 2 divided doses

**Drugs to avoid in pregnancy**
ACE inhibitors, ARBs, direct renin inhibitors — Angiotensin converting enzyme (ACE) inhibitors, angiotensin II receptor blockers (ARBs) and direct renin inhibitors are contraindicated at all stages of pregnancy

## 23.5 BP target in treatment of HTN disease in pregnancy

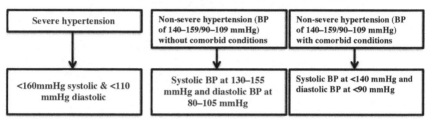

| BP target in treatment of HTN disease in pregnancy | | |
|---|---|---|
| Severe hypertension | Non-severe hypertension (BP of 140–159/90–109 mmHg) without comorbid conditions | Non-severe hypertension (BP of 140–159/90–109 mmHg) with comorbid conditions |
| <160mmHg systolic & <110 mmHg diastolic | Systolic BP at 130–155 mmHg and diastolic BP at 80–105 mmHg | Systolic BP at <140 mmHg and diastolic BP at <90 mmHg |

## 23.6 Time of delivery in chronic HTN patient

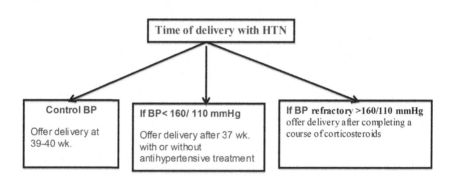

| Time of delivery with HTN | | |
|---|---|---|
| **Control BP** <br> Offer delivery at 39-40 wk. | **If BP< 160/ 110 mmHg** <br> Offer delivery after 37 wk. with or without antihypertensive treatment | **If BP refractory >160/110 mmHg** <br> offer delivery after completing a course of corticosteroids |

# 23.7 Post partum follow up with chronic HTN

Referral to a specialist in hypertensive disorders in-patient with secondary chronic    HTN

-Measure BP daily for the first 2 days after birth, then every 3 days for 1 wks Aiming to keep blood pressure lower than 140/90 mmHg.

**Post partum medication** hydralazine, labetalol, nifedipine, & methyldopa are safe with breast-feeding

Resume preconception antihypertensive treatment

Prefer to medical team 6-8 wks posy partum

## 23.8   Gestational hypertension classification

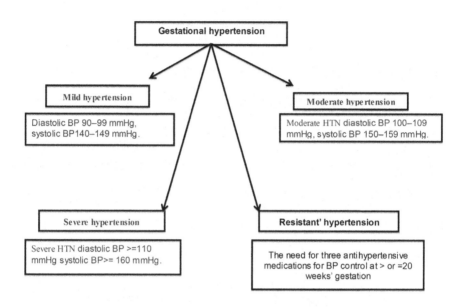

```
                  ┌─────────────────────────────┐
                  │  Gestational hypertension   │
                  └─────────────────────────────┘
```

**Mild hypertension**

Diastolic BP 90–99 mmHg,
systolic BP140–149 mmHg.

**Moderate hypertension**

Moderate HTN diastolic BP 100–109
mmHg, systolic BP 150–159 mmHg.

**Severe hypertension**

Severe HTN diastolic BP >=110
mmHg systolic BP>= 160 mmHg.

**Resistant' hypertension**

The need for three antihypertensive
medications for BP control at > or =20
weeks' gestation

## 23.9   Gestational hypertension

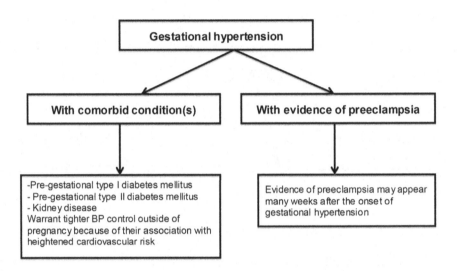

## 23.10   Management of pregnancy with gestational HTN

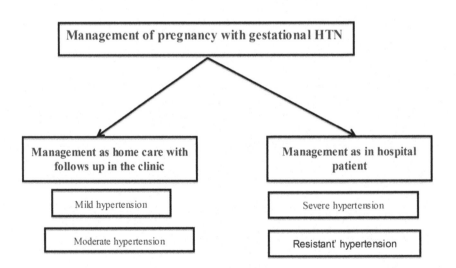

# 23.11 Preconception advice

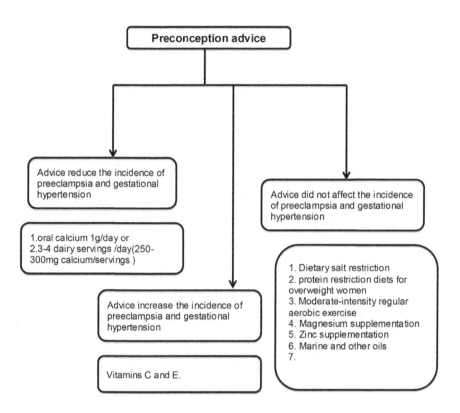

Preconception advice

Advice reduce the incidence of preeclampsia and gestational hypertension

1.oral calcium 1g/day or
2.3-4 dairy servings /day(250-300mg calcium/servings )

Advice increase the incidence of preeclampsia and gestational hypertension

Vitamins C and E.

Advice did not affect the incidence of preeclampsia and gestational hypertension

1. Dietary salt restriction
2. protein restriction diets for overweight women
3. Moderate-intensity regular aerobic exercise
4. Magnesium supplementation
5. Zinc supplementation
6. Marine and other oils
7.

# 23.12  ANC follow up of patient with gestational hypertension

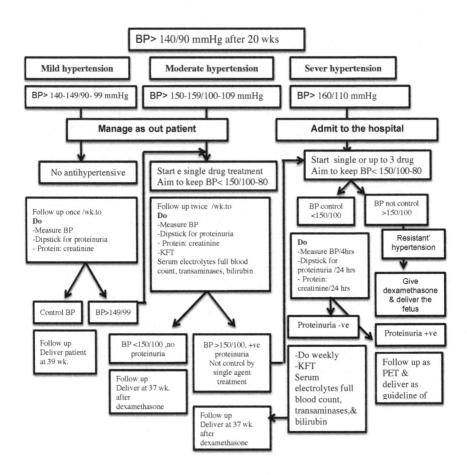

BP> 140/90 mmHg after 20 wks

| Mild hypertension | Moderate hypertension | Sever hypertension |
|---|---|---|
| BP> 140-149/90- 99 mmHg | BP> 150-159/100-109 mmHg | BP> 160/110 mmHg |

**Manage as out patient**

**Admit to the hospital**

No antihypertensive

Start e single drug treatment
Aim to keep BP< 150/100-80

Start single or up to 3 drug
Aim to keep BP< 150/100-80

Follow up once /wk.to
**Do**
-Measure BP
-Dipstick for proteinuria
- Protein: creatinine

Follow up twice /wk.to
**Do**
-Measure BP
-Dipstick for proteinuria
- Protein: creatinine
-KFT
Serum electrolytes full blood
count, transaminases, bilirubin

BP control
<150/100

BP not control
>150/100

Resistant'
hypertension

**Do**
-Measure BP/4hrs
-Dipstick for
proteinuria /24 hrs
- Protein:
creatinine/24 hrs

Give
dexamethasone
& deliver the
fetus

Control BP

BP>149/99

Proteinuria -ve

Proteinuria +ve

Follow up
Deliver patient
at 39 wk.

BP <150/100 ,no
proteinuria

BP >150/100, +ve
proteinuria
Not control by
single agent
treatment

-Do weekly
-KFT
Serum
electrolytes full
blood count,
transaminases,&
bilirubin

Follow up as
PET &
deliver as
guideline of

Follow up
Deliver at 37 wk.
after
dexamethasone

Follow up
Deliver at 37 wk.
after
dexamethasone

# 23.13   Time of delivery

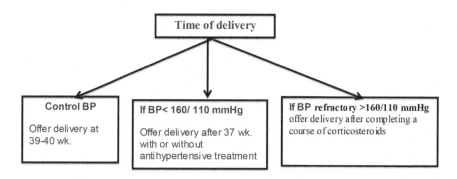

Time of delivery

**Control BP**

Offer delivery at 39-40 wk.

**If BP< 160/ 110 mmHg**

Offer delivery after 37 wk. with or without antihypertensive treatment

**If BP refractory >160/110 mmHg** offer delivery after completing a course of corticosteroids

## 23.14 Postnatal investigation, monitoring and treatment

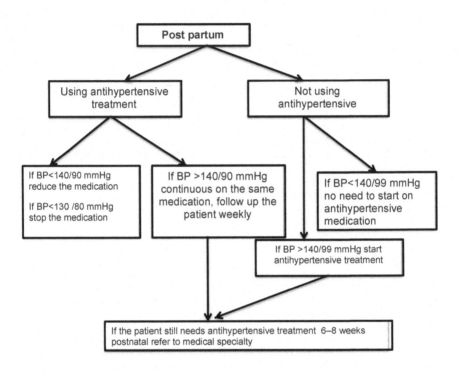

Post partum

Using antihypertensive treatment

Not using antihypertensive

If BP<140/90 mmHg reduce the medication

If BP<130 /80 mmHg stop the medication

If BP >140/90 mmHg continuous on the same medication, follow up the patient weekly

If BP<140/99 mmHg no need to start on antihypertensive medication

If BP >140/99 mmHg start antihypertensive treatment

If the patient still needs antihypertensive treatment 6–8 weeks postnatal refer to medical specialty

If patient on methyldopa stop within 2 days after birth

# 24   Protein S deficiency

**Protein S deficiency**

**Hereditary**

- Autosomal dominant trait. Thrombosis is observed in both heterozygous (2% incompatible with life ) and homozygous genetic deficiencies of protein S.

-Protein S and C levels are lower in sickle cell anemia and they decrease further significantly during crisis

**Acquired**

Is usually due to
- Hepatic diseases
-   vitamin K deficiency
-   result of antagonism with oral warfarin anticoagulants
-   low levels of protein S in pregnancy do not cause thrombosis by themselves.
-   Disseminated intravascular coagulation
-   HIV infection
-   The nephrotic syndrome
-   Age affects total protein S but not free protein S levels
-   Patient recover from chickenpox

## 24.1 Management of protein S deficiency

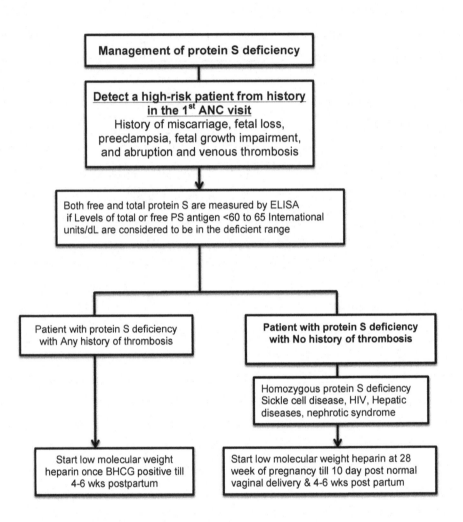

Management of protein S deficiency

**Detect a high-risk patient from history in the 1st ANC visit**
History of miscarriage, fetal loss, preeclampsia, fetal growth impairment, and abruption and venous thrombosis

Both free and total protein S are measured by ELISA if Levels of total or free PS antigen <60 to 65 International units/dL are considered to be in the deficient range

Patient with protein S deficiency with Any history of thrombosis

**Patient with protein S deficiency with No history of thrombosis**

Homozygous protein S deficiency Sickle cell disease, HIV, Hepatic diseases, nephrotic syndrome

Start low molecular weight heparin once BHCG positive till 4-6 wks postpartum

Start low molecular weight heparin at 28 week of pregnancy till 10 day post normal vaginal delivery & 4-6 wks post partum

# 25   Systemic lupus erythematosus

# 25.1   Clinical course of SLE in pregnancy

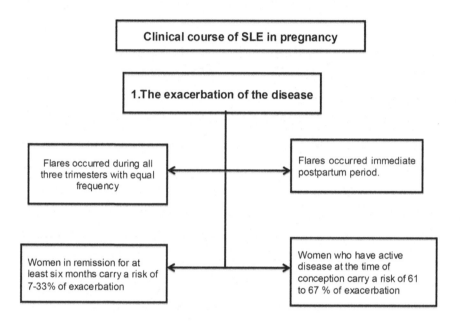

## 25.2 The exacerbation of renal disease in SLE patient

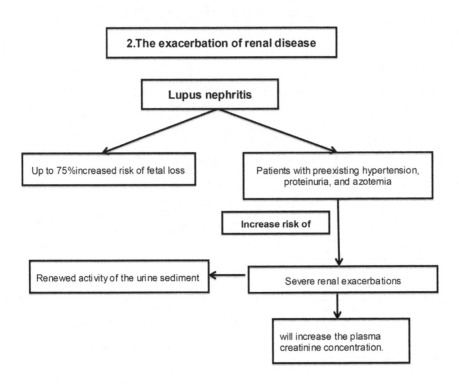

2.The exacerbation of renal disease

Lupus nephritis

Up to 75%increased risk of fetal loss

Patients with preexisting hypertension, proteinuria, and azotemia

Increase risk of

Renewed activity of the urine sediment

Severe renal exacerbations

will increase the plasma creatinine concentration.

## 25.3 Pregnancy following renal transplantation

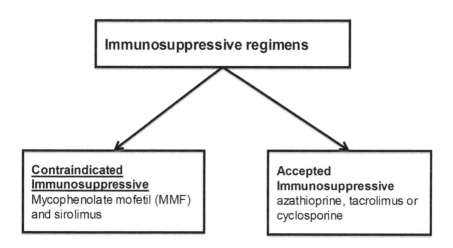

**Immunosuppressive regimens**

**Contraindicated Immunosuppressive**
Mycophenolate mofetil (MMF) and sirolimus

**Accepted Immunosuppressive**
azathioprine, tacrolimus or cyclosporine

## 25.4 Treatment of patient with SLE Recommendation

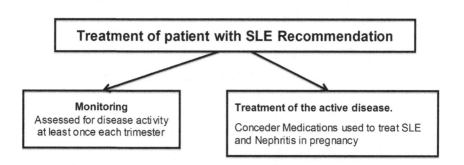

**Treatment of patient with SLE Recommendation**

**Monitoring**
Assessed for disease activity at least once each trimester

**Treatment of the active disease.**
Conceder Medications used to treat SLE and Nephritis in pregnancy

## 25.5   ANC follow up for patient with SLE

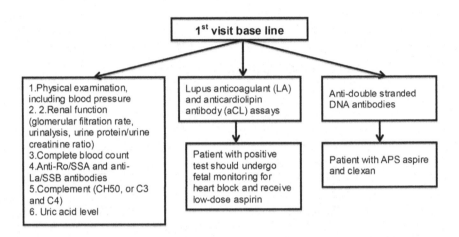

| 1ˢᵗ visit base line |

**1.Physical examination,** including blood pressure
2. 2.Renal function (glomerular filtration rate, urinalysis, urine protein/urine creatinine ratio)
3.Complete blood count
4.Anti-Ro/SSA and anti-La/SSB antibodies
5.Complement (CH50, or C3 and C4)
6. Uric acid level

Lupus anticoagulant (LA) and anticardiolipin antibody (aCL) assays

Patient with positive test should undergo fetal monitoring for heart block and receive low-dose aspirin

Anti-double stranded DNA antibodies

Patient with APS aspire and clexan

# 25.6   Monitoring of SLE patient in the last trimester

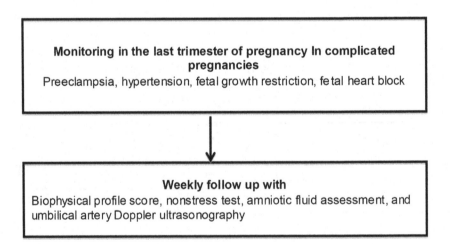

**Monitoring in the last trimester of pregnancy In complicated pregnancies**
Preeclampsia, hypertension, fetal growth restriction, fetal heart block

**Weekly follow up with**
Biophysical profile score, nonstress test, amniotic fluid assessment, and umbilical artery Doppler ultrasonography

## 25.7 Management of patient with SLE in the postpartum period

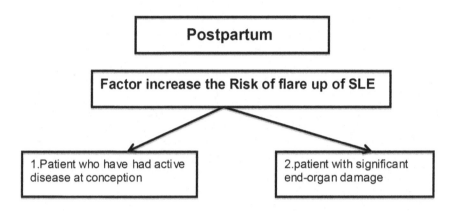

Postpartum

Factor increase the Risk of flare up of SLE

1.Patient who have had active disease at conception

2.patient with significant end-organ damage

## 25.8 Drug safe for the nursing infant

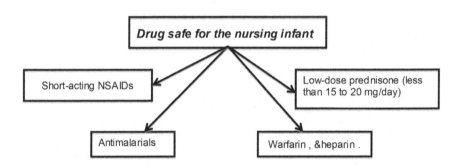

*Drug safe for the nursing infant*

Short-acting NSAIDs

Low-dose prednisone (less than 15 to 20 mg/day)

Antimalarials

Warfarin , &heparin .

# 25.9    Treatment of active disease.

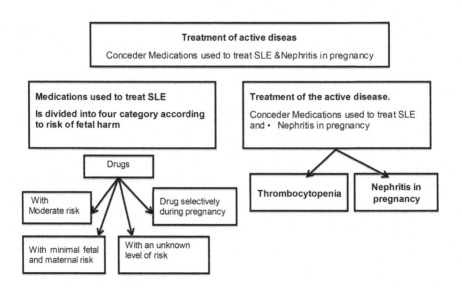

# 25.10    Drug with Moderate to high risk of fetal harm

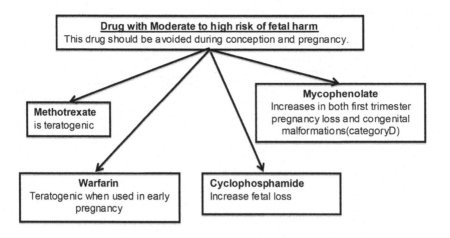

# 25.11 Drug with Minimal fetal and maternal risk

**Drug with Minimal fetal and maternal risk**
NSAID use during early and late pregnancy and antimalarial drug use throughout pregnancy are probably safe.

**NSAIDs**
NSAIDs are safe during the latter part of the first and during the second trimester but should be discontinued in the last trimester of pregnancy.

**Antimalarial drugs**
The safety of drugs is uncertain, Patients who discontinue hydroxychloroquine prior to, or during, pregnancy are more likely to have exacerbations of SLE

**Unknown level of risk**

Use of biologic antirheumatic drugs such as B cell targeted antibodies (e.g., rituximab ) and T-B cell costimulation blockers (e.g. abatacept) is discouraged in part because of a lack of data on safety of their use during pregnancy.

# 25.12   Drug with Selective use allowed during pregnancy

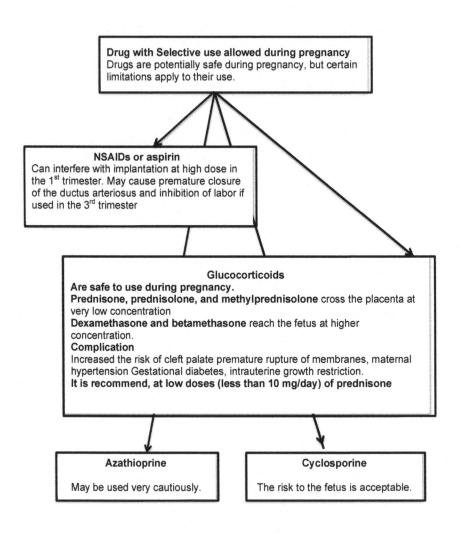

**Drug with Selective use allowed during pregnancy**
Drugs are potentially safe during pregnancy, but certain limitations apply to their use.

**NSAIDs or aspirin**
Can interfere with implantation at high dose in the 1$^{st}$ trimester. May cause premature closure of the ductus arteriosus and inhibition of labor if used in the 3$^{rd}$ trimester

**Glucocorticoids**
**Are safe to use during pregnancy.**
**Prednisone, prednisolone, and methylprednisolone** cross the placenta at very low concentration
**Dexamethasone and betamethasone** reach the fetus at higher concentration.
**Complication**
Increased the risk of cleft palate premature rupture of membranes, maternal hypertension Gestational diabetes, intrauterine growth restriction.
**It is recommend, at low doses (less than 10 mg/day) of prednisone**

**Azathioprine**

May be used very cautiously.

**Cyclosporine**

The risk to the fetus is acceptable.

# 25.13   Thrombocytopenia in SLE

**Thrombocytopenia**

During lupus pregnancies may have multiple causes

Thrombocytopenia can be due to Antiplatelet antibodies, toxemia, and antiphospholipid antibodies. Treatment includes high-dose prednisone and intravenous immune globulin

# 26   Pregnancy with kidney disease

# 26.1   Preconception advice for effect of pregnancy on kidney disease

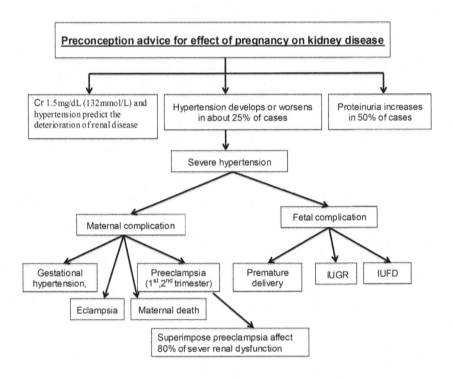

# 26.2   Effect of pregnancy on renal function RF

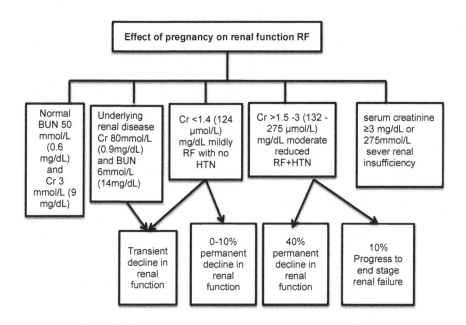

Effect of pregnancy on renal function RF

- Normal BUN 50 mmol/L (0.6 mg/dL) and Cr 3 mmol/L (9 mg/dL)
- Underlying renal disease Cr 80mmol/L (0.9mg/dL) and BUN 6mmol/L (14mg/dL)
- Cr <1.4 (124 µmol/L) mg/dL mildly RF with no HTN
- Cr >1.5 -3 (132 - 275 µmol/L) mg/dL moderate reduced RF+HTN
- serum creatinine ≥3 mg/dL or 275mmol/L sever renal insufficiency

- Transient decline in renal function
- 0-10% permanent decline in renal function
- 40% permanent decline in renal function
- 10% Progress to end stage renal failure

## 26.3  Management of pregnant women with renal disease

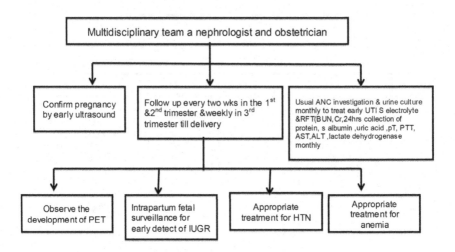

Multidisciplinary team a nephrologist and obstetrician

Confirm pregnancy by early ultrasound

Follow up every two wks in the 1st &2nd trimester &weekly in 3rd trimester till delivery

Usual ANC investigation & urine culture monthly to treat early UTI S electrolyte &RFT(BUN,Cr,24hrs collection of protein, s albumin ,uric acid ,pT, PTT, AST,ALT ,lactate dehydrogenase monthly

Observe the development of PET

Intrapartum fetal surveillance for early detect of IUGR

Appropriate treatment for HTN

Appropriate treatment for anemia

# 26.4   Special situation in pregnancy with renal disease

## Patient with renal transplant

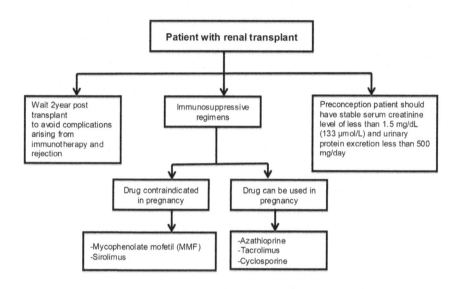

**Patient with renal transplant**

Wait 2year post transplant to avoid complications arising from immunotherapy and rejection

Immunosuppressive regimens

Preconception patient should have stable serum creatinine level of less than 1.5 mg/dL (133 µmol/L) and urinary protein excretion less than 500 mg/day

Drug contraindicated in pregnancy

Drug can be used in pregnancy

-Mycophenolate mofetil (MMF)
-Sirolimus

-Azathioprine
-Tacrolimus
-Cyclosporine

# Patient with Intensive dialysis

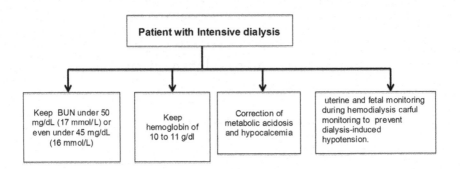

**Patient with Intensive dialysis**

Keep BUN under 50 mg/dL (17 mmol/L) or even under 45 mg/dL (16 mmol/L)

Keep hemoglobin of 10 to 11 g/dl

Correction of metabolic acidosis and hypocalcemia

uterine and fetal monitoring during hemodialysis carful monitoring to prevent dialysis-induced hypotension.

# 27 Rh and other blood group alloimmunizations

# 27.1 Follow up of Rh-negative blood group

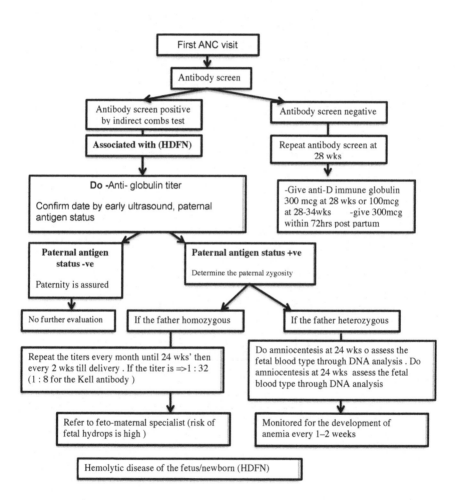

First ANC visit

Antibody screen

Antibody screen positive by indirect combs test

**Associated with (HDFN)**

Antibody screen negative

Repeat antibody screen at 28 wks

**Do -Anti- globulin titer**

Confirm date by early ultrasound, paternal antigen status

-Give anti-D immune globulin 300 mcg at 28 wks or 100mcg at 28-34wks    -give 300mcg within 72hrs post partum

**Paternal antigen status -ve**

Paternity is assured

**Paternal antigen status +ve**

Determine the paternal zygosity

No further evaluation

If the father homozygous

If the father heterozygous

Repeat the titers every month until 24 wks' then every 2 wks till delivery . If the titer is =>1 : 32 ( 1 : 8 for the Kell antibody )

Do amniocentesis at 24 wks o assess the fetal blood type through DNA analysis . Do amniocentesis at 24 wks  assess the fetal blood type through DNA analysis

Refer to feto-maternal specialist (risk of fetal hydrops is high )

Monitored for the development of anemia every 1–2 weeks

Hemolytic disease of the fetus/newborn (HDFN)

## 27.2　ANC follow up and Monitored for the development of fetal anemia

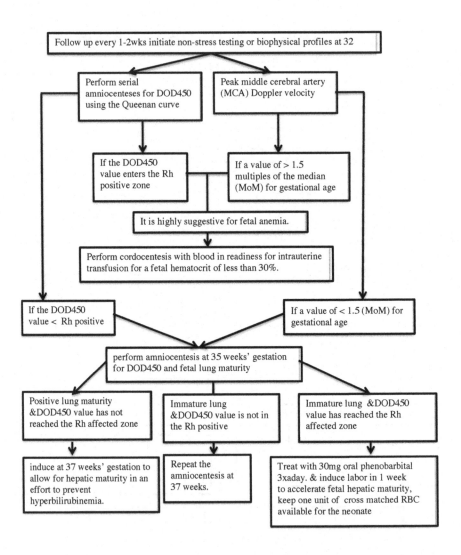

Follow up every 1-2wks initiate non-stress testing or biophysical profiles at 32

Perform serial amniocenteses for DOD450 using the Queenan curve

Peak middle cerebral artery (MCA) Doppler velocity

If the DOD450 value enters the Rh positive zone

If a value of > 1.5 multiples of the median (MoM) for gestational age

It is highly suggestive for fetal anemia.

Perform cordocentesis with blood in readiness for intrauterine transfusion for a fetal hematocrit of less than 30%.

If the DOD450 value < Rh positive

If a value of < 1.5 (MoM) for gestational age

perform amniocentesis at 35 weeks' gestation for DOD450 and fetal lung maturity

Positive lung maturity &DOD450 value has not reached the Rh affected zone

Immature lung &DOD450 value is not in the Rh positive

Immature lung &DOD450 value has reached the Rh affected zone

induce at 37 weeks' gestation to allow for hepatic maturity in an effort to prevent hyperbilirubinemia.

Repeat the amniocentesis at 37 weeks.

Treat with 30mg oral phenobarbital 3xaday. & induce labor in 1 week to accelerate fetal hepatic maturity, keep one unit of cross matched RBC available for the neonate

## 27.3   Management of subsequent Alloimmune pregnancy

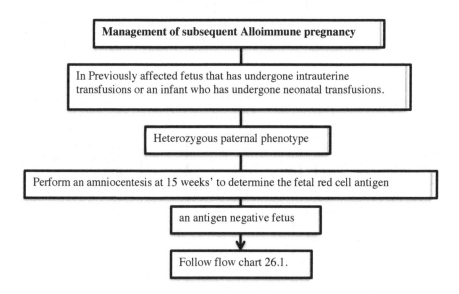

Management of subsequent Alloimmune pregnancy

In Previously affected fetus that has undergone intrauterine transfusions or an infant who has undergone neonatal transfusions.

Heterozygous paternal phenotype

Perform an amniocentesis at 15 weeks' to determine the fetal red cell antigen

an antigen negative fetus

Follow flow chart 26.1.

# 28.  Epilepsy in pregnancy

# 28.1  Preconception advice

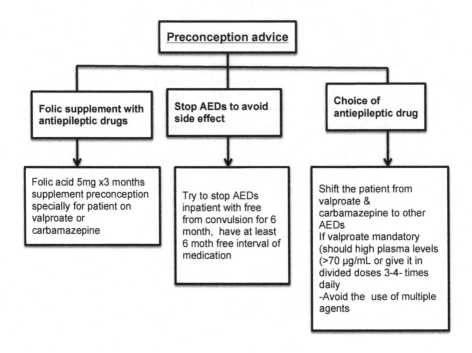

**Preconception advice**

**Folic supplement with antiepileptic drugs**

Folic acid 5mg x3 months supplement preconception specially for patient on valproate or carbamazepine

**Stop AEDs to avoid side effect**

Try to stop AEDs inpatient with free from convulsion for 6 month, have at least 6 moth free interval of medication

**Choice of antiepileptic drug**

Shift the patient from valproate & carbamazepine to other AEDs
If valproate mandatory (should high plasma levels (>70 µg/mL or give it in divided doses 3-4- times daily
-Avoid the use of multiple agents

# 28.2   Management of epileptic patient during pregnancy

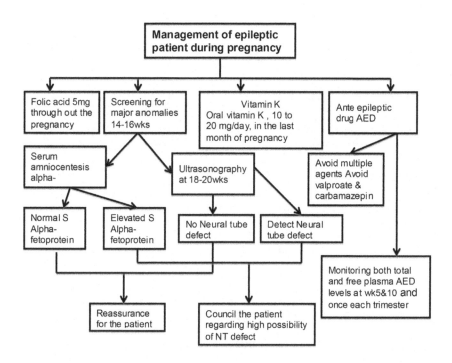

# 28.3 Mode of delivery in patient with epilepsy

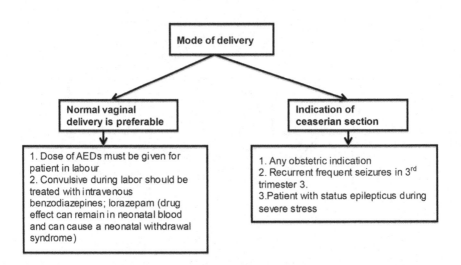

Mode of delivery

Normal vaginal delivery is preferable

1. Dose of AEDs must be given for patient in labour
2. Convulsive during labor should be treated with intravenous benzodiazepines; lorazepam (drug effect can remain in neonatal blood and can cause a neonatal withdrawal syndrome)

Indication of ceaserian section

1. Any obstetric indication
2. Recurrent frequent seizures in 3rd trimester 3.
3. Patient with status epilepticus during severe stress

# 28.4 Post partum care for patient with epilepsy

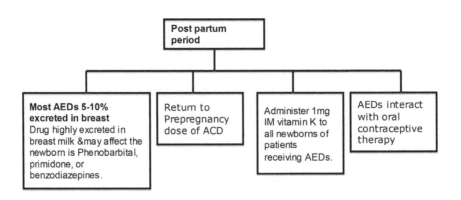

Post partum period

Most AEDs 5-10% excreted in breast
Drug highly excreted in breast milk &may affect the newborn is Phenobarbital, primidone, or benzodiazepines.

Return to Prepregnancy dose of ACD

Administer 1mg IM vitamin K to all newborns of patients receiving AEDs.

AEDs interact with oral contraceptive therapy

# 29  Cardiac disease in pregnancy

# 29.1  type of cardiac diseas in pregnancy

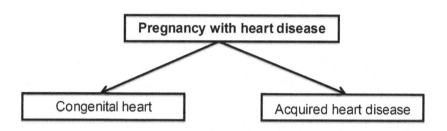

| Pregnancy with heart disease |
| --- |

**Congenital heart**

1.trial septal defect (ASD)
2. Ventricular septal defect (VSD)
3.unrepaired tetralogy of Fallot
4.pulmonary atresia with aorto-pulmonary collaterals
5. Single ventricular lesions
6. Tricuspid atresia
7. Ebstein's anomaly with right-to-left shunts via an ASD
8. Congenitally corrected transposition of the great arteries with VSD or ASD

**Acquired heart disease**

1.Poor functional class class II to IV) or cyanosis
2.Previous cardiac event (eg, heart failure, transient ischemic attack, stroke) or arrhythmia
3.Left heart obstruction (mitral valve area of <2 cm2, aortic valve area of <1.5 cm2, peak left ventricular outflow gradient >30 mmHg)
4.Left ventricular systolic dysfunction (left ventricular ejection fraction <40 percent)

# 29.2 Condition associated with maternal and fetal risk

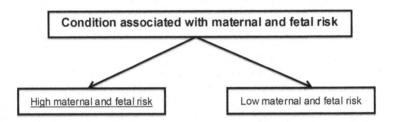

| High maternal and fetal risk | Low maternal and fetal risk |
|---|---|
| 1. Severe aortic stenosis with or without symptoms<br>2.Symptomatic mitral stenosis (NYHA class II to IV)<br>3.Aortic or mitral regurgitation with NYHA class III to IV symptoms<br>4.Aortic and/or mitral valve disease with severe left ventricular dysfunction (LVEF < 40 %) or severe pulmonary hypertension (pulmonary artery pressure >75 %of systemic pressure)<br>5.Marfan syndrome with or without aortic regurgitation<br>6.Mechanical prosthetic valve requiring anticoagulation | 1.Asymptomatic aortic stenosis with an LVEF >50 percent and a mean gradient < 25 mmHg<br>2.Aortic or mitral regurgitation with no or mild symptoms (NYHA class I to II)<br>3.Mitral valve prolapse with either no mitral regurgitation or mild to moderate mitral regurgitation with an LVEF >50 percent<br>4.Mild mitral stenosis (defined as a mitral valve area >1.5 cm2 and a mean gradient less the 5 mmHg) without severe pulmonary hypertension (pulmonary artery pressure >75 percent of systemic pressure)<br>5.Mild to moderate pulmonary valve stenosis |

Cardiac surgery should be avoided during pregnancy due to high risk on the fetus for the fetus, no difference in the maternal risk .

## 29.3    ANC for patient with cardiac disease

```
┌─────────────────────────────────────────────────┐
│       ANC for patient with cardiac disease        │
└─────────────────────────────────────────────────┘
         ↙                              ↘
┌──────────────────────┐      ┌──────────────────────┐
│  Maternal monitoring  │      │    Fetal monitoring    │
└──────────────────────┘      └──────────────────────┘
         ↓                              ↓
```

| Maternal monitoring | Fetal monitoring |
|---|---|
| 1.Identify and treat any factor that can deteriorate cardiac function (anemia, infection, arrhythmia, or non-physiologic edema)<br><br>2. Limit the physical activity for patient with cyanotic ventricular dysfunction functional class III or IV<br><br>3.close monitoring in the 3$^{rd}$ trimester | 1.Monitor fetal development<br>2.Do perform fetal echocardiogram performed between 18 and 22<br><br>3.close monitoring for fetal development in the 3$^{rd}$ trimmest twice weekly |

# 29.4   Mode of delivery in cardiac patient

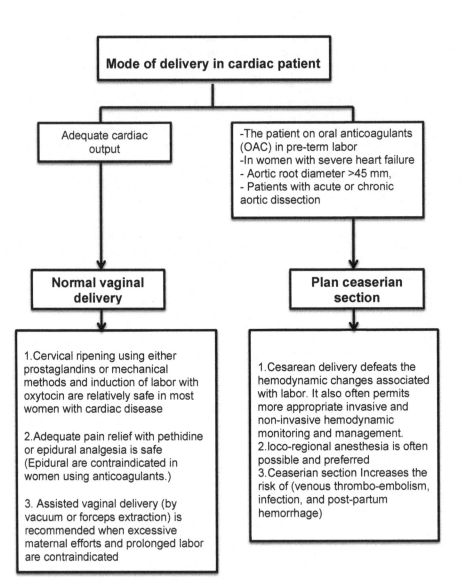

Mode of delivery in cardiac patient

Adequate cardiac output

-The patient on oral anticoagulants (OAC) in pre-term labor
-In women with severe heart failure
- Aortic root diameter >45 mm,
- Patients with acute or chronic aortic dissection

**Normal vaginal delivery**

**Plan ceaserian section**

1.Cervical ripening using either prostaglandins or mechanical methods and induction of labor with oxytocin are relatively safe in most women with cardiac disease

2.Adequate pain relief with pethidine or epidural analgesia is safe (Epidural are contraindicated in women using anticoagulants.)

3. Assisted vaginal delivery (by vacuum or forceps extraction) is recommended when excessive maternal efforts and prolonged labor are contraindicated

1.Cesarean delivery defeats the hemodynamic changes associated with labor. It also often permits more appropriate invasive and non-invasive hemodynamic monitoring and management.
2.loco-regional anesthesia is often possible and preferred
3.Ceaserian section Increases the risk of (venous thrombo-embolism, infection, and post-partum hemorrhage)

# Section II Instruction manual in Labour room

# 30 Diagnoses and Management of patient in Labor

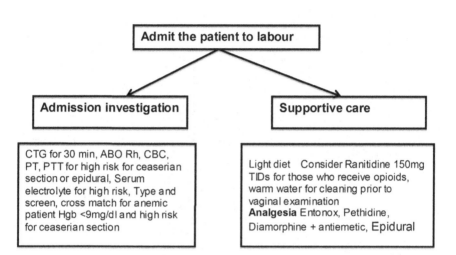

Admit the patient to labour

Admission investigation

CTG for 30 min, ABO Rh, CBC, PT, PTT for high risk for ceaserian section or epidural, Serum electrolyte for high risk, Type and screen, cross match for anemic patient Hgb <9mg/dl and high risk for ceaserian section

Supportive care

Light diet    Consider Ranitidine 150mg TIDs for those who receive opioids, warm water for cleaning prior to vaginal examination
**Analgesia** Entonox, Pethidine, Diamorphine + antiemetic, Epidural

# 30.1 Patient assessment in emergency room

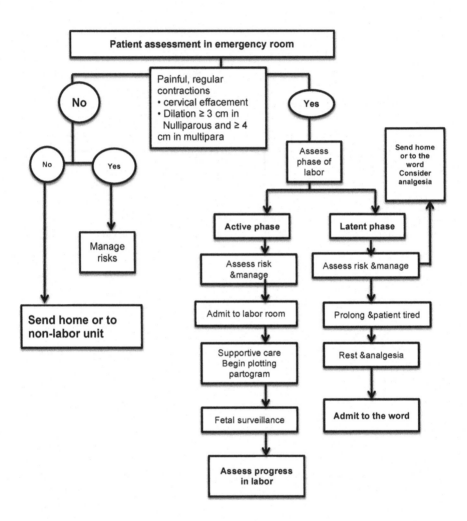

# 30.2　Patient assessment in labor room

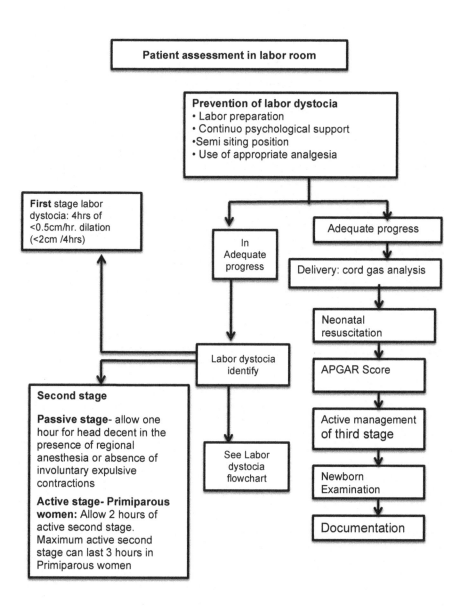

Patient assessment in labor room

**Prevention of labor dystocia**
• Labor preparation
• Continuo psychological support
•Semi siting position
• Use of appropriate analgesia

**First** stage labor dystocia: 4hrs of <0.5cm/hr. dilation (<2cm /4hrs)

In Adequate progress

Adequate progress

Delivery: cord gas analysis

Neonatal resuscitation

APGAR Score

Labor dystocia identify

**Second stage**

**Passive stage**- allow one hour for head decent in the presence of regional anesthesia or absence of involuntary expulsive contractions

**Active stage- Primiparous women:** Allow 2 hours of active second stage. Maximum active second stage can last 3 hours in Primiparous women

See Labor dystocia flowchart

Active management of third stage

Newborn Examination

Documentation

# 30.3   Third Stage of Labor

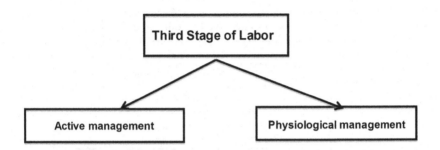

**Third Stage of Labor**

**Active management**

**Physiological management**

1.Average length is 30 minutes
2. Give 5 "u" oxytocin IM or slow Intravenously **OR** Syntometrine 500 microgram / 5 IU synthetic oxytocin OR Methergin (0.4 mg intramuscular) with the delivery of anterior shoulder
3. Delivery of the placenta should be done by the midwife/obstetrician conducted the delivery by controlled cord traction within two minutes after administration of Oxytocin and Syntometrine.

2.Average length is 60 minutes Wait for the sign of separation of placenta (prolongation of the cord, gush of blood and ascending of the uterus

# 30.4   Category of the CTG

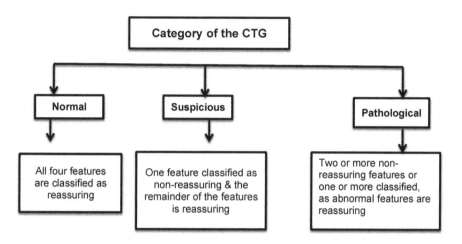

---

**Essential practical point for Performing Electronic Fetal Monitoring (EFM))**

- The date and time on the EFM machine should be correctly set, ensure machine is set to 1cm/hour.

- The cardiotocograph label should be used to record mother's name, date of birth and hospital number, maternal pulse rate, reason for EFM, date and time of trace commenced, signature of midwife.

- Any antenatal/intrapartum events that may affect the FH rate should be noted contemporaneously on the CTG and in the maternal notes, signed  and the date and time noted (VE's, FBS sampling, siting of an epidural)•

# 30.5 Categorization of Fetal Heart Rate

| Feature | Baseline (b/pm) | Variability (b/pm) | Decelerations |
|---|---|---|---|
| Reassuring | 110-160 | >5 | None |
| Non-reassuring | 161–180 | Less than 5 for 30–90 minutes | Variable decelerations: Dropping from baseline by 60 beats/ minute or less and taking 60 seconds or less to recover Present for over 90 minutes Occurring with over 50% of contractions. **OR** Variable decelerations: Dropping from baseline by more than 60 beats/ minute or taking over 60 seconds to recover present for up to 30 minutes occurring with over 50% of contractions. **OR** Late decelerations: present for up to 30 minutes Occurring with over 50% of contractions |

| Abnormal | Above 180 Or below 100 | Less than 5 for over 90 minutes | Non-reassuring variable decelerations (see row above): still observed 30 minutes after starting conservative measures occurring with over 50% of contractions. OR Late decelerations: present for over 30 minutes Do not improve with conservative measures Occurring with over 50% of contractions. OR Bradycardia or a single prolonged deceleration lasting 3 minutes or more. |
|---|---|---|---|

# 30.6 Management of CTG:

| Category | Definition | Interpretation | Management |
|---|---|---|---|
| CTG is normal/ reassuring | All 3 features are normal/ reassuring | Normal CTG, no non-reassuring or abnormal features, healthy fetus | Continue CTG and normal care. If CTG was started because of concerns Arising from intermittent auscultation, Remove CTG after 20 minutes if there are no non-reassuring or abnormal features and no ongoing risk factors. |

| CTG is non-reassuring and suggests need for conservative measures | 1 non-reassuring feature AND 2 normal/ reassuring features | Combination of features that may be associated with increased risk of fetal acidosis; if accelerations are present, acidosis is unlikely | Think about possible underlying causes. If the baseline fetal heart rate is over 160 beats/ minute, Check the woman's temperature and pulse. If either are raised, offer fluids & paracetamol. Start 1 or more conservative measures: Encourage the woman to mobilise or adopt a left-lateral position,& in particular To avoid being supine offer oral or intravenous fluids reduce contraction frequency by stopping oxytocin if being used and/or offering tocolysis. Inform coordinating midwife & obstetrician. |

| CTG is abnormal and indicates need for conservative measures AND further testing | 1 abnormal feature OR 2 non-reassuring features | Combination of features that is more likely to be associated with fetal acidosis | CTG is abnormal and indicates need for conservative Measures AND further testing 1 abnormal feature OR 2 non-reassuring features Combination of features that is more likely to be associated with fetal acidosis Discuss with the consultant obstetrician if an FBS cannot be obtained or a third FBS is thought to be needed. |
|---|---|---|---|

| | | | |
|---|---|---|---|
| CTG is abnormal and indicates need for urgent intervention | Bradycardia or a single prolonged deceleration with baseline below 100 beats/ minute, persisting for 3 minutes or more* | An abnormal feature that is very likely to be associated with current fetal acidosis or imminent rapid development of fetal acidosis | Start 1 or more conservative measures (See 'CTG is non-reassuring...' row for details). Inform coordinating midwife. Urgently seek obstetric help. Make preparations for urgent birth. Expedite birth if persists for 9 minutes. If heart rate recovers before 9 minutes, Reassess decision to expedite birth in discussion With the woman. |

---

**Abbreviations: CTG, cardiotocograph; FBS, fetal blood sample.**

A stable baseline value of 90–99 beats/minute with normal baseline variability (having confirmed that this is not the maternal heart rate) may be a normal variation; obtain a senior obstetric opinion if uncertain.

**The presence of fetal heart rate accelerations is generally a sign that the baby is healthy; the absence of accelerations in an otherwise normal cardiotocograph trace does not indicate**

# 30.7   Classification of Fetal Blood Sample Results

| FETAL pH | SUBSEQUENT ACTION |
|----------|-------------------|
| >/=7.25 | Repeat FBS within 1 hour if the FHR remains pathological |
| 7.21-7.24 | Repeat FBS within 30 minutes if the FHR remains pathological or consider Delivery if rapid fall since the last sample |
| </=7.20 | Delivery indicated |

# 31   Regimen for Syntocinon Infusion

## Regimen A Primigravida

*10 unit oxytocin in 500 ml 1 mile international Unit =3ml micro drop/min(3ml/hrs)

| MiliInternational unit/min | Micro drop/min (mL/hr.) |
|---|---|
| 2 | 6 |
| 4 | 12 |
| 6 | 18 |
| 8 | 24 |
| 10 | 30 |
| 12 | 36 |
| 14 | 42 |
| 16 | 48 |
| 18 | 54 |
| 20 | 60 |
| 22 | 66 |
| 24 | 72 |
| 26 | 78 |
| 28 | 84 |
| 30 | 90 |
| 32 | 96 |
| 34 | 102 |
| 36 | 108 |
| 38 | 114 |
| 40 | 120 |

**Regimen B Multigravida** *10 unit oxytocin in 500 ml 1 mile international Unit =3ml micro drop/min(3ml/hrs)

| Mili International unit/min | Micro drop/min (mL/hr.) |
|---|---|
| 1 | 3 |
| 2 | 6 |
| 3 | 9 |
| 4 | 12 |
| 5 | 15 |
| 6 | 18 |
| 7 | 21 |
| 8 | 24 |
| 9 | 27 |
| 10 | 30 |
| 11 | 33 |
| 12 | 36 |
| 13 | 39 |
| 14 | 42 |
| 15 | 45 |
| 16 | 48 |
| 17 | 51 |
| 18 | 54 |
| 19 | 57 |
| 20 | 60 |
| 21 | 63 |
| 22 | 66 |
| 23 | 69 |
| 24 | 72 |
| 25 | 75 |
| 26 | 78 |
| 27 | 81 |

| | |
|---|---|
| 28 | 84 |
| 29 | 87 |
| 30 | 90 |
| 31 | 93 |
| 32 | 96 |
| 33 | 99 |
| 34 | 102 |
| 35 | 105 |
| 36 | 108 |

*Syntocinon should not be started for six hours following administration of vaginal prostaglandins gel and half an hour after Propess.*

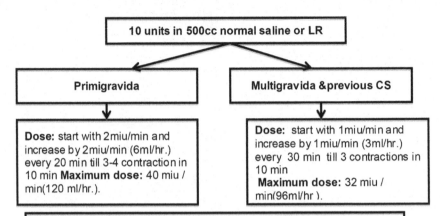

**10 units in 500cc normal saline or LR**

**Primigravida**

**Multigravida &previous CS**

**Dose:** start with 2miu/min and increase by 2miu/min (6ml/hr.) every 20 min till 3-4 contraction in 10 min **Maximum dose:** 40 miu / min(120 ml/hr.).

**Dose:** start with 1miu/min and increase by 1miu/min (3ml/hr.) every 30 min till 3 contractions in 10 min
**Maximum dose:** 32 miu / min(96ml/hr ).

If hyper stimulation or CTG abnormalities occur a, Stop Syntocinon, give I.V. infusion, tocolysis.

# 32   Cord Blood Sampling

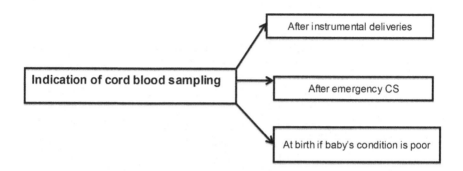

Indication of cord blood sampling

After instrumental deliveries

After emergency CS

At birth if baby's condition is poor

**Procedure**:   Double clamp umbilical cord, collect paired samples from the umbilical artery and umbilical vein either with a pre-heparinized syringe or a pre-heparinized tube. NB: the specimen remains stable at room temperature for up to 1 hour.   **Interpretation:**   Lower limit of normal may range from 7.02 - 7.18 but the risk of mortality and morbidity does not increase unless the value is < 7.00 and even then the risk is small.

**Values of <7.1 should be reported**

**Cases with ph<7.1 with BD>10 should be audited**

# 33  Guidelines for the care of women' presenting in labor

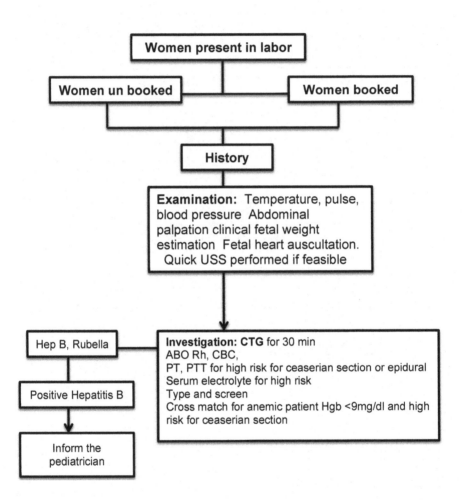

# 34   Group B Streptococcus (GBS) in Labor

# 34.1   Prevention of Perinatal Group B Streptococcal (GBS) Disease

**Intrapartum antibiotic prophylaxis (IAP) is recommended for:**

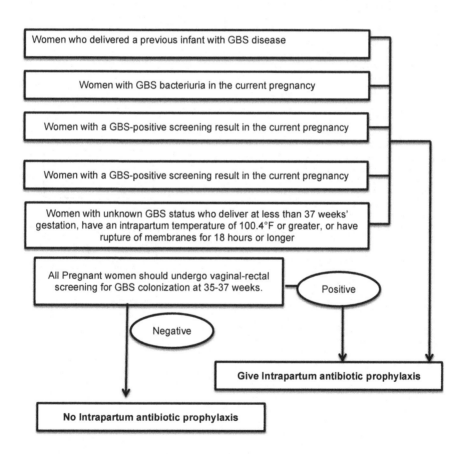

Women who delivered a previous infant with GBS disease

Women with GBS bacteriuria in the current pregnancy

Women with a GBS-positive screening result in the current pregnancy

Women with a GBS-positive screening result in the current pregnancy

Women with unknown GBS status who deliver at less than 37 weeks' gestation, have an intrapartum temperature of 100.4°F or greater, or have rupture of membranes for 18 hours or longer

All Pregnant women should undergo vaginal-rectal screening for GBS colonization at 35-37 weeks.

Positive

Negative

Give Intrapartum antibiotic prophylaxis

No Intrapartum antibiotic prophylaxis

# 34.2 Recommended regimens for intrapartum antibiotic prophylaxis for prevention of early-onset group B streptococcal (GBS) disease

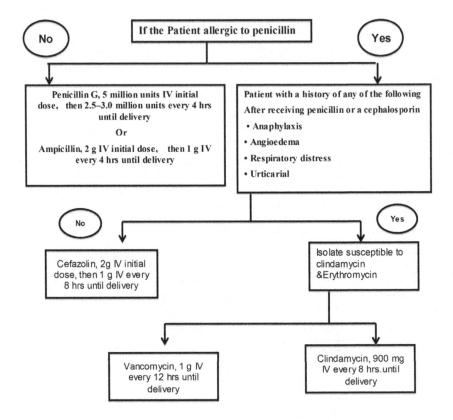

## 34.3   Group B Streptococcus(GBS) in Labor Pathway

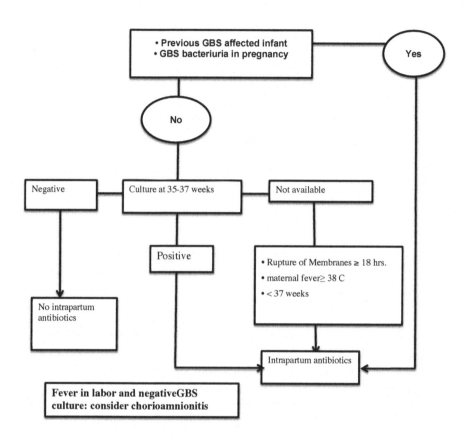

# 35   Induction of Labor (IOL)

## Indication for induction of labor

1. Preeclampsia ≥ 37 weeks

2. Significant maternal disease not responding to treatment

3. Significant but stable antepartum hemorrhage

4. Chorioamnionitis

5. Suspected fetal compromise

6. Term pre-labour rupture of membranes with maternal GBS colonization    Postdates (> 41+0 weeks) or post-term (> 42+0 weeks) pregnancy.

**Relative indication for induction**

-Uncomplicated twin pregnancy ≥ 38 weeks

-Diabetes mellitus (glucose control may dictate urgency)

-Alloimmune disease at or near term

-Intrauterine growth restriction

-Oligohydramnios

-Gestational hypertension ≥ 38 weeks

-Intrauterine fetal death

-PROM at or near term, GBS negative

-Logistical problems (history of rapid labour, distance to hospital)

-Intrauterine death in a prior pregnancy (Induction may be performed to alleviate parental anxiety, but there is no known medical or outcome advantage for mother or baby.

-SLE at 38 wks.

## Contraindication

1. Placenta or vasa previa or cord presentation

2. Abnormal fetal lie or presentation (e.g. transverse lie or footling breech)

3. Prior classical or inverted T uterine incision

4. Significant prior uterine surgery (e.g. full thickness myomectomy)

5. Active genital herpes

6. Pelvic structural deformities

Placenta or vasa previa or cord presentation

• Abnormal fetal lie or presentation (e.g. transverse lie or footling breech)

• Prior classical or inverted T uterine incision

• significant prior uterine surgery (e.g. full thickness myomectomy)

• Active genital herpes

• Pelvic structural deformities

## Unacceptable indications

1. Care provider or patient convenience

2. Suspected fetal macrosomia (estimated fetal weight   > 4000 gm.) in a non-diabetic women is an unacceptable indication because there is no reduction in the incidence of shoulder dystocia but twice the risk of CS.

# 35.1 Defention needed in induction of labor

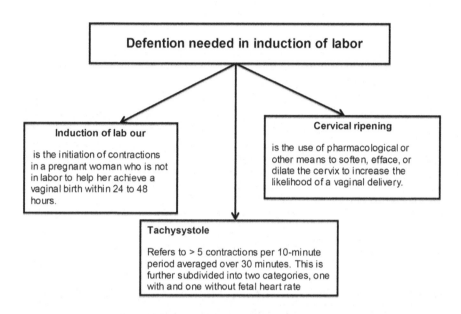

Defention needed in induction of labor

**Induction of lab our**

is the initiation of contractions in a pregnant woman who is not in labor to help her achieve a vaginal birth within 24 to 48 hours.

**Cervical ripening**

is the use of pharmacological or other means to soften, efface, or dilate the cervix to increase the likelihood of a vaginal delivery.

**Tachysystole**

Refers to > 5 contractions per 10-minute period averaged over 30 minutes. This is further subdivided into two categories, one with and one without fetal heart rate

**Factors influence the success rates of induction :** Bishop score, parity (prior vaginal delivery), BMI, maternal age, estimated fetal weight, and diabetes changes

# 35.2 Modified Bishop Scoring System

Score

| Factor | 0 | 1 | 2 |
|---|---|---|---|
| Dilatation/cm | 0 | 1-2 | 3-4 |
| Effacement, % | 0-30 | 40-50 | 60-70 |
| Length, cm | >3 | 1-3 | <1 |
| Consistency | firm | medium | Soft |
| Position | Posterior | mid | Anterior |
| Station | Sp-3or above | Sp-2 | Sp-1 or0 |

**A favorable pre- induction Bishop score of > 6 are predictive of a successful vaginal delivery.**

1. Health care providers should assess the cervix (using the Bishop score) to determine the likelihood of success and to select the appropriate method of induction.

# 35.3 Ripening / induction: of unfavorable Cervix

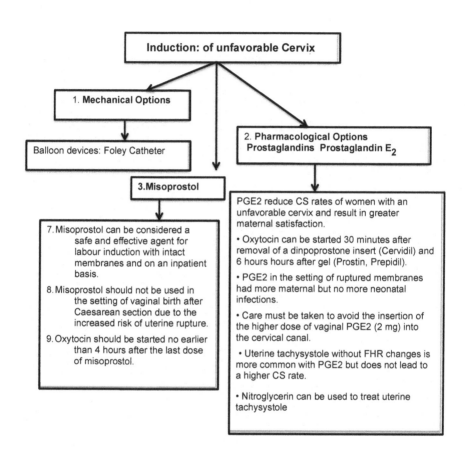

Induction: of unfavorable Cervix

1. Mechanical Options

Balloon devices: Foley Catheter

2. Pharmacological Options
Prostaglandins  Prostaglandin E$_2$

3. Misoprostol

7. Misoprostol can be considered a safe and effective agent for labour induction with intact membranes and on an inpatient basis.

8. Misoprostol should not be used in the setting of vaginal birth after Caesarean section due to the increased risk of uterine rupture.

9. Oxytocin should be started no earlier than 4 hours after the last dose of misoprostol.

PGE2 reduce CS rates of women with an unfavorable cervix and result in greater maternal satisfaction.

• Oxytocin can be started 30 minutes after removal of a dinpoprostone insert (Cervidil) and 6 hours hours after gel (Prostin, Prepidil).

• PGE2 in the setting of ruptured membranes had more maternal but no more neonatal infections.

• Care must be taken to avoid the insertion of the higher dose of vaginal PGE2 (2 mg) into the cervical canal.

• Uterine tachysystole without FHR changes is more common with PGE2 but does not lead to a higher CS rate.

• Nitroglycerin can be used to treat uterine tachysystole

# 35.4    Induction With a Favorable Cervix

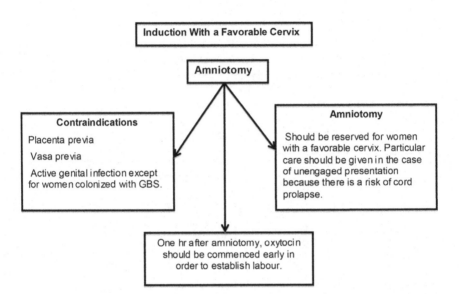

Induction With a Favorable Cervix

Amniotomy

**Contraindications**

Placenta previa

Vasa previa

Active genital infection except for women colonized with GBS.

**Amniotomy**

Should be reserved for women with a favorable cervix. Particular care should be given in the case of unengaged presentation because there is a risk of cord prolapse.

One hr after amniotomy, oxytocin should be commenced early in order to establish labour.

# 35.5   Induction of labor pathway

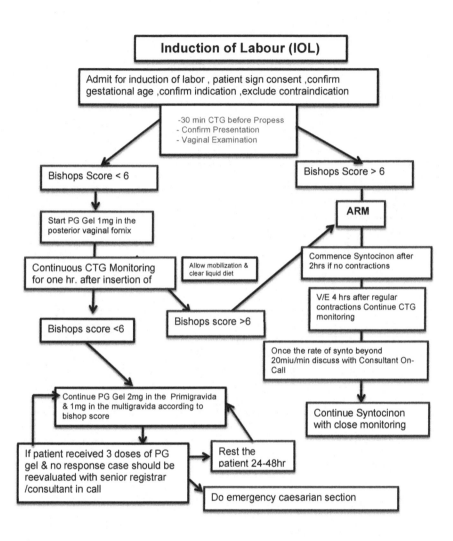

**Induction of Labour (IOL)**

Admit for induction of labor , patient sign consent ,confirm gestational age ,confirm indication ,exclude contraindication

-30 min CTG before Propess
- Confirm Presentation
- Vaginal Examination

Bishops Score < 6

Bishops Score > 6

Start PG Gel 1mg in the posterior vaginal fornix

**ARM**

Continuous CTG Monitoring for one hr. after insertion of

Allow mobilization & clear liquid diet

Commence Syntocinon after 2hrs if no contractions

V/E 4 hrs after regular contractions Continue CTG monitoring

Bishops score <6

Bishops score >6

Once the rate of synto beyond 20miu/min discuss with Consultant On-Call

Continue PG Gel 2mg in the  Primigravida & 1mg in the multigravida according to bishop score

Continue Syntocinon with close monitoring

If patient received 3 doses of PG gel & no response case should be reevaluated with senior registrar /consultant in call

Rest the patient 24-48hr

Do emergency caesarian section

# 36 The Management of Third- and Fourth-Degree Perineal Tears

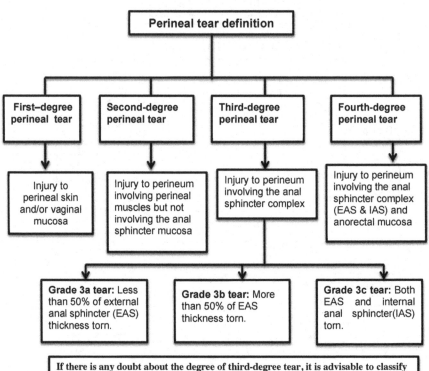

**Perineal tear definition**

| First–degree perineal tear | Second-degree perineal tear | Third-degree perineal tear | Fourth-degree perineal tear |

Injury to perineal skin and/or vaginal mucosa

Injury to perineum involving perineal muscles but not involving the anal sphincter mucosa

Injury to perineum involving the anal sphincter complex

Injury to perineum involving the anal sphincter complex (EAS & IAS) and anorectal mucosa

**Grade 3a tear:** Less than 50% of external anal sphincter (EAS) thickness torn.

**Grade 3b tear:** More than 50% of EAS thickness torn.

**Grade 3c tear:** Both EAS and internal anal sphincter(IAS) torn.

If there is any doubt about the degree of third-degree tear, it is advisable to classify it to the higher degree rather than the lower degree.

# 36.1 Repair of third- and fourth-degree pathway

Obstetric anal sphincter repair should be performed by consultant /senior registrar who's well train in repair

Repair should take place in an operating theatre, under regional or general anesthesia, with good lighting and with appropriate instruments.

In case of excessive bleeding, a vaginal pack should be inserted

For repair of a full thickness external anal sphincter (EAS) tear, either an overlapping or an end-to- end (approximation) method can be used with equivalent outcomes.

The torn anorectal mucosa should be repaired with 3-0 polyglactin sutures using either the continuous or interrupted technique.

The torn internal anal sphincter (IAS) can be identified, &repair separately with interrupted or mattress 3-0 PDS or 2-0 polyglactin sutures without any attempt to overlap the IAS

For partial thickness (all 3a and some 3b) tears, an end-to-end technique should be used.

The use of broad-spectrum IV antibiotics for 48hr follow by oral antibiotics for 1wk &the use of postoperative laxatives for one wk

Follow up for reevaluation 6-12wk-post partum for reevaluation

# 37 Labor Management of women with previous Caesarean Section in

## 37.1 Planned vaginal birth after ceaserian section

Vaginal birth after ceaserian section

**Contraindications to VBAC**

1. Women with previous uterine rupture or classical caesarean scar

2. women who have other absolute contraindications to vaginal birth that applies irrespective of the presence or absence of a scar (e.g. major placenta praevia).

3. women with complicated uterine scars, caution should be exercised and decisions should be made on a case-by-case basis by a senior obstetrician with access to the details of previous surgery.

**Planned VBAC**

Can be offered to a women with a singleton pregnancy with cephalic presentation at $37^{+0}$ weeks or beyond who have had a single previous lower segment caesarean delivery, with or without a history of previous vaginal birth.

Women who have had two or more prior lower segment caesarean deliveries may be offered VBAC after counseling by a senior obstetrician. This should include the risk of uterine rupture and maternal morbidity, and the individual likelihood of successful VBAC (e.g. given a history of prior vaginal delivery).

# 37.2 Labor &birth in previous Ceaserian section

| Labor &birth in previous CS | 1. Labour is managed to optimize a normal outcome |
| | 2. Delivery planned at labor room with availability of obstetric theatre and onsite blood transfusion |
| | 3. IV Access with ABO and Group & Save samples sent |
| | 4 One to one care with midwife |
| | 5. Continuous CTG monitoring (Fetal distress has been reported to precede uterine rupture) |
| | 6. Meticulous monitoring of progress of labour. |
| | 7. Concerns with progress of labour should be reported to registrar on call for labour ward. |
| | 8. The use of Syntocinon to augment poor progress or secondary arrest must be discussed with the consultant |
| | 9. Guideline for the use of Syntocinon in VBAC is identical to the guidelines for its use with any other labour |
| | 10. Epidural analgesia is available on request |
| | 11. Regular maternal observations including BP, Pulse and temperature |

**Awareness of classical symptoms of scar rupture - pain, scar tenderness, bleeding PV, maternal tachycardia, hypotension and fetal distress**

**Post partum scar palpation not required.**

## 37.3   Induction of labor in VBAC pathway1

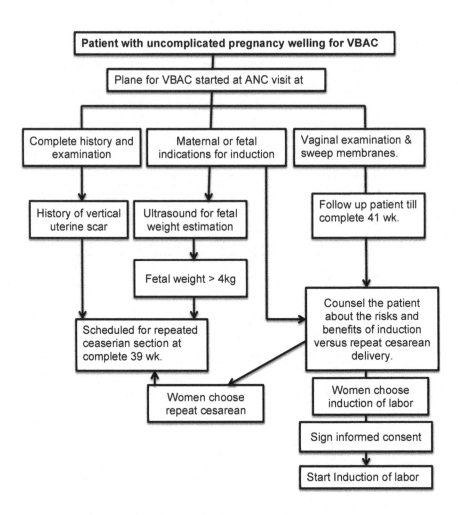

# 37.4 Unfavorable cervix

## Induction in Unfavorable cervix previous CS

### Single balloon catheter

-Under aseptic technique can use the # 16 foly catheter with balloon

Do continuous uterine activity monitoring.

Ring forceps can be used to pass a deflated balloon bladder catheter then inflate it with 60 mL NS ) through the internal cervical os and into the extra amniotic space. The balloon is retracted so that it rests against the internal os.

The catheter is left in place until it is extruded or for up to 12 hours.

-Oxytocin is begun after the catheter has been extruded or removed.

A large balloon catheter may be more effective than a small one.

### Intravaginal prostaglandins E2 gel

1mg every 6 hrs. for 3 doses the to be reevaluated with senior registrar/consultant on duty if not responding

Intra-vaginal prostaglandins are preferred to intra-cervical prostaglandins E2 because they results in more timely vaginal deliveries.

# 37.5   Favorable cervix

Induction of Favorable cervix in previous CS

Cervical ripening is unnecessary
Start with amniotomy and administration of oxytocin
A low-dose infusion oxytocin typically consists of an initial dose
between 0.5 and 2.0-mill units/min, increase every 30 min till 3
regular contraction in 10 min maximumdose 32 miu

Misoprostol is not advice for induction in preveous ceaserian section

# 37.6 Induction of labor in previous scar pathway2

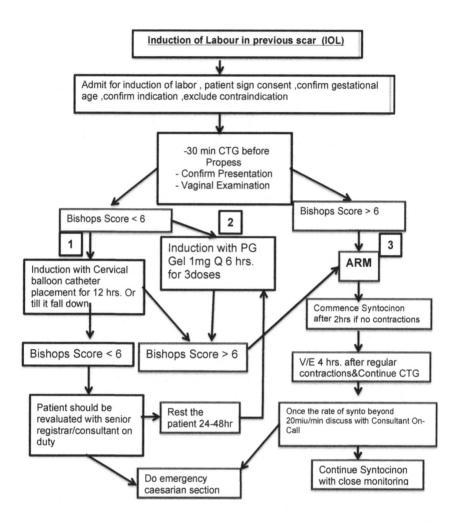

**Induction of Labour in previous scar (IOL)**

Admit for induction of labor , patient sign consent ,confirm gestational age ,confirm indication ,exclude contraindication

-30 min CTG before Propess
- Confirm Presentation
- Vaginal Examination

Bishops Score < 6

Bishops Score > 6

**2**

**1**

Induction with Cervical balloon catheter placement for 12 hrs. Or till it fall down

Induction with PG Gel 1mg Q 6 hrs. for 3doses

**3**

**ARM**

Commence Syntocinon after 2hrs if no contractions

Bishops Score < 6

Bishops Score > 6

V/E 4 hrs. after regular contractions&Continue CTG

Patient should be revaluated with senior registrar/consultant on duty

Rest the patient 24-48hr

Once the rate of synto beyond 20miu/min discuss with Consultant On-Call

Continue Syntocinon with close monitoring

Do emergency caesarian section

# 38   Spontaneous Ruptures
# OF Membranes (SROM)


# 38.1   Diagnosis


| Diagnosis |
|---|
| 1. If frank leaking no need for speculum examination<br>2. If it is uncertain do speculum examination<br>3. Avoid digital vaginal examination in the absence of contractions. |

# 38.2  Management of SROM>37wks

## Immediate IOL

If the patient develop any of

1. Chorioamnionitis

2. Antenatal history of GBS

3. Signs of fetal compromise

4. Maternal request (depends on labour ward occupancy)

- The risk of serious neonatal infection is 1%, rather than 0.5% for women with intact membranes
- 60% of women with Prelabour rupture of the membranes will go into labour within 24 hours

## Expectant Management

1. Patient allowed to go home with information sheet, thermometer to record temperature

2. To check temperature at home 4 hourly during working waking hours 3.If temperature >37°c or unwell, to return to hospital IOL - in 24hrs

Prophylactic antibiotics as per guideline

- No need for lower vaginal swabs and measurement of maternal Creative protein
- Monitor for the development of infection by record the temperature every 4 hours and report any change in the color or smell of the vaginal loss, reduce fetal movement or abdominal tenderness

# 38.3   Spontaneous rupture of membrane (PPROM)<37wks pathway

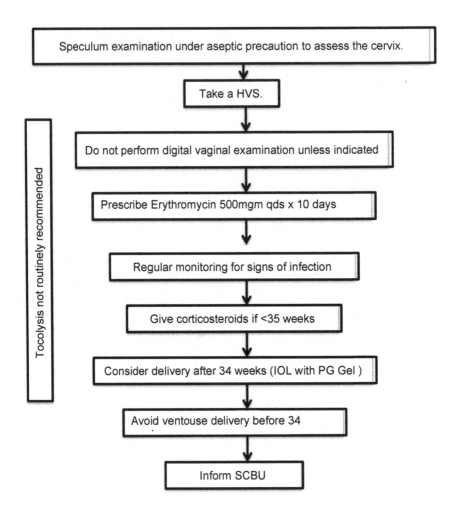

Speculum examination under aseptic precaution to assess the cervix.

Take a HVS.

Do not perform digital vaginal examination unless indicated

Prescribe Erythromycin 500mgm qds x 10 days

Regular monitoring for signs of infection

Give corticosteroids if <35 weeks

Consider delivery after 34 weeks (IOL with PG Gel )

Avoid ventouse delivery before 34

Inform SCBU

Tocolysis not routinely recommended

# 39    PRE-TERMLABOUR

# 39.1    Defention of preterm labour

## Definition of preterm labour

Pre-term is birth of a baby less than 37 weeks of gestation age. Associated with Painful uterine contractions occurring >1 in 10 mints with cervical effacement &dilatation.

# 39.2    Initial assessment

## Initial assessment Threatened pre-term/pre-term labour

Pulse, temperature,

BP, urine dipstick/MSU

CTG monitoring

CBC, group & save

Abdominal exam

Scan for presentation

Speculum exam for cervical dilatation

Vaginal exam if only indicated

# 39.3   Pre term labor guidline

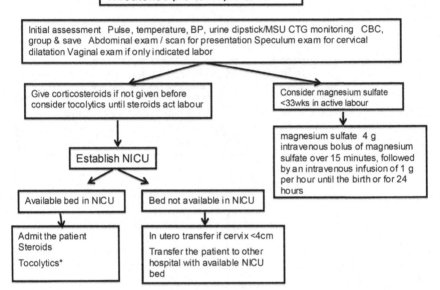

Threatened pre-term/pre-term

Initial assessment  Pulse, temperature, BP, urine dipstick/MSU CTG monitoring   CBC, group & save   Abdominal exam / scan for presentation Speculum exam for cervical dilatation Vaginal exam if only indicated labor

Give corticosteroids if not given before consider tocolytics until steroids act labour

Consider magnesium sulfate <33wks in active labour

magnesium sulfate  4 g intravenous bolus of magnesium sulfate over 15 minutes, followed by an intravenous infusion of 1 g per hour until the birth or for 24 hours

Establish NICU

Available bed in NICU

Bed not available in NICU

Admit the patient
Steroids

Tocolytics*

In utero transfer if cervix <4cm

Transfer the patient to other hospital with available NICU bed

# 40   Corticosteroids

1.Antenatal Corticosteroids given to Reduce Neonatal Morbidity & Mortality

# 40.1   Indication for administration of corticosteroids

1.all women at risk of iatrogenic or spontaneous preterm birth up to 34+6 weeks of gestation.

2. all women booked for an elective caesarean section prior to 38+6 weeks of gestation.

3.donot give  prophylactic steroids in women with a previous history of preterm delivery or multiple pregnancies who show no signs of being at risk of preterm birth.

4.donot give  corticosteroids at gestations <24+0 weeks unless you discuss it counsultant obstetric and neonatologist

5.Antenatal corticosteroids are most effective in reducing RDS in patient deliver 24 hours after and up to 7 days after administration of the second dose of antenatal corticosteroids.

6.No reduction in neonatal death, RDS or cerebroventricular hemorrhage is seen in infants delivered more than 7 days after treatment with antenatal corticosteroids.

7.if the intial course of cortecosteriod given before 26 wks second dose can be given after the opinion of counsultant on duty

# 40.2   Administration of corticosteroid in special situation

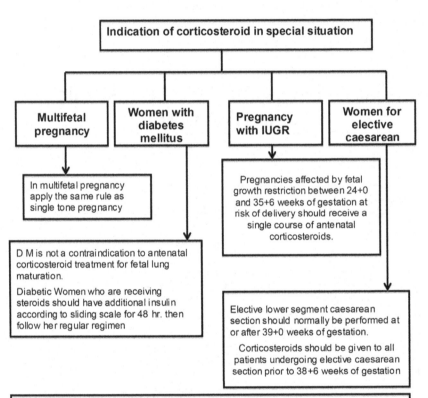

**Indication of corticosteroid in special situation**

**Multifetal pregnancy**

**Women with diabetes mellitus**

**Pregnancy with IUGR**

**Women for elective caesarean**

In multifetal pregnancy apply the same rule as single tone pregnancy

Pregnancies affected by fetal growth restriction between 24+0 and 35+6 weeks of gestation at risk of delivery should receive a single course of antenatal corticosteroids.

D M is not a contraindication to antenatal corticosteroid treatment for fetal lung maturation.

Diabetic Women who are receiving steroids should have additional insulin according to sliding scale for 48 hr. then follow her regular regimen

Elective lower segment caesarean section should normally be performed at or after 39+0 weeks of gestation.

Corticosteroids should be given to all patients undergoing elective caesarean section prior to 38+6 weeks of gestation

**Contraindications to the use of antenatal corticosteroids**

Caution should be exercised when giving to women with systemic infection including tuberculosis or sepsis.

**Senior opinion** should be taken when contemplating delaying delivery for steroid prophylaxis in cases of overt chorioamnionitis.

## 40.3   Type, dose administration corticosteroids

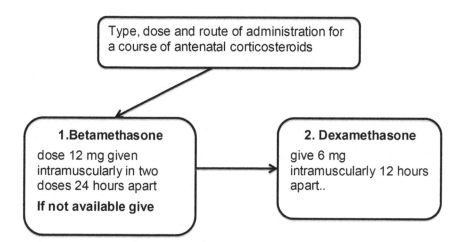

Type, dose and route of administration for a course of antenatal corticosteroids

**1.Betamethasone**

dose 12 mg given intramuscularly in two doses 24 hours apart

**If not available give**

**2. Dexamethasone**

give 6 mg intramuscularly 12 hours apart..

# 41   Tocolytics

Should be considered to complete a course of steroids or in utero transfer in case of preterm

**First drug of choice**

Nifedipine regime – 20 mgm of oral Nifedipine as loading dose-followed

by 10- 20mgm three to four times daily, adjusted according to uterine activity up to 48hrs (total dose of 60mgm) labour
**\*After giving nifedipine-loading dose please check the pulse rate and BP every 30 minutes for first 2 hours then 4 hourly until next dose**

| Contraindication | Relative Contraindication |
|---|---|

- Cardiogenic shock & Aortic stenosis
- Severe PET
- Intrauterine infection
- Placental abruption
- Advanced cervical dilatation
- Evidence of fetal compromise

  Placental insufficiency

- Non reassuring CTG
- IUGR
- Multiple pregnancy

  Mild hemorrhage due to placenta previa

# 41.1   Atosiban

*The choice of Atosiban (licensed) should be discussed with the duty Consultant.*

| Step | Regimen | Injection Rate | Atosiban dose |
|------|---------|----------------|---------------|
| Bolus | Over 1 min | 0.9 ml. | 6.75 mg |
| Loading dose | 3 hours | 24 ml/hour | 18 mg/hour (300 mcg/ min) |
| Maintenance dose | Up to 45 hours | 8 ml/hour | 6 mg/hour (100 mcg/ min) |

Atosiban

**Preparation**

Atosiban = Tractocile = 7.5mg/ml   Infusion can be given in 0.9% saline, Ringer solution, or 5% Dextrose

From a 100 ml bag, withdraw 10 ml and discard, replace it with 10 ml s Atosiban 7.5 mg/ml=75 mg in 100ml.

Loading infusion 24ml/hour=18mg/hour over 3 hours then reduce the infusion rate to 8ml/hour

☐No specific antidote

**Contraindications to Atosiban**

>33 wks., <24 wks.,

☐PROM>30 wks.

☐Abnormal FH

☐Placenta previa, abruption

☐Severe Pre eclampsia

No data on women with abnormal liver or renal function

Theoretically increase of ph.

☐No effect on lactation

☐No specific antidote

# 42 Hypertensive disease in pregnancy

## 42.1 Definitions of HTN disease in pregnancy

| Hypertensive disease in pregnancy |
| --- |

| Mild Hypertension | Severe hypertension |
| --- | --- |
| BP 140-149/90-99 mmHg | BP ≥ 160/110 mmHg with multisystem involvement |

| Aim of the therapy is to keep BP < 150/80-100 mmHg |
| --- |

# 42.2   Preeclampsia definition

```
┌─────────────────────────────────────────────────────────┐
│              Definitions of preeclampsia                 │
│  New-onset hypertension (systolic blood pressure >=140 mm Hg │
│  or diastolic blood pressure >90 mm Hg) and new-onset    │
│  proteinuria after 20 weeks' gestation in a previously   │
│  normotensive patient                                    │
└─────────────────────────────────────────────────────────┘
```

| Mil preeclampsia | Sever preeclampsia |
|---|---|
| BP >140/90<br>Proteinuria >300mg<br>No multisystem involvement | BP >160/110<br>Thrombocytopenia &<br>multisystem involvement |

| Hypertension | Proteinuria | Multisystem Involvement |
|---|---|---|
| >140 mm Hg systolic or >90 mm Hg diastolic | >300 mg in 24 h | Thrombocytopenia |
| Previously normotensive patient >20 wk. gestation | Protein/creatinine ratio >=0.3 mg/dl | Renal insufficiency |
| BP measured two times at least 4 hours apart | Dipstick 11 (only if other methods not available) | Liver dysfunction |
|  |  | Pulmonary edema |
|  |  | Cerebral or visual disturbances |

# 42.3  Preeclampsia management pathway

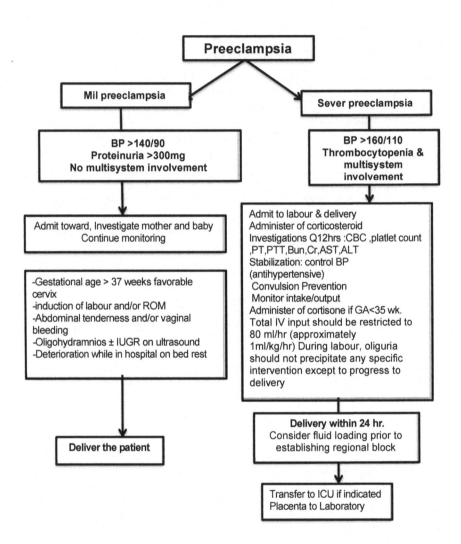

# 42.4   Features of Severe preeclampsia

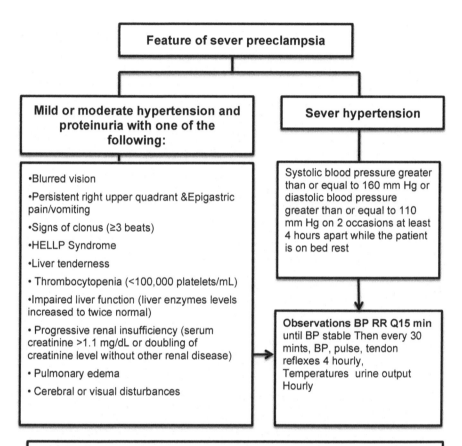

**Feature of sever preeclampsia**

**Mild or moderate hypertension and proteinuria with one of the following:**

•Blurred vision

•Persistent right upper quadrant &Epigastric pain/vomiting

•Signs of clonus (≥3 beats)

•HELLP Syndrome

•Liver tenderness

• Thrombocytopenia (<100,000 platelets/mL)

•Impaired liver function (liver enzymes levels increased to twice normal)

• Progressive renal insufficiency (serum creatinine >1.1 mg/dL or doubling of creatinine level without other renal disease)

• Pulmonary edema

• Cerebral or visual disturbances

**Sever hypertension**

Systolic blood pressure greater than or equal to 160 mm Hg or diastolic blood pressure greater than or equal to 110 mm Hg on 2 occasions at least 4 hours apart while the patient is on bed rest

**Observations BP RR Q15 min** until BP stable Then every 30 mints, BP, pulse, tendon reflexes 4 hourly, Temperatures  urine output Hourly

**Continuous fetal monitoring Restrict fluid 80ml/hr Episodically ausculate the chest, optic fundi  Follow Pathway for postnatal management of PET/Eclamps**

# 43   Eclampsia

## 43.1   Eclampsia management pathway

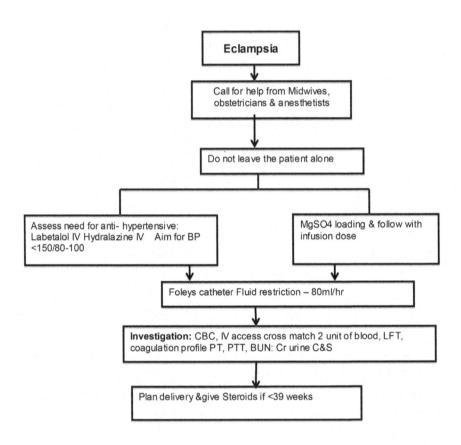

## 43.2   Recurrence of seizures management pathway

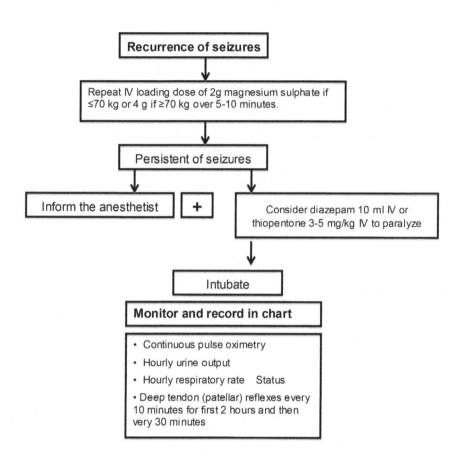

Recurrence of seizures

Repeat IV loading dose of 2g magnesium sulphate if ≤70 kg or 4 g if ≥70 kg over 5-10 minutes.

Persistent of seizures

Inform the anesthetist

**+**

Consider diazepam 10 ml IV or thiopentone 3-5 mg/kg IV to paralyze

Intubate

Monitor and record in chart

- Continuous pulse oximetry
- Hourly urine output
- Hourly respiratory rate    Status
- Deep tendon (patellar) reflexes every 10 minutes for first 2 hours and then very 30 minutes

**Stop magnesium sulphate infusion and check the levels**

**If**

Urine output is < 100 ml in 4 hours

- Patellar reflexes are absent (assuming not due to regional block)

- Respiratory rate < 16 beats/ minute

- $O_2$ saturation is < 90% There is no need to measure magnesium levels if urine output is maintained Check magnesium levels if toxicity is suspected on clinical grounds

**The antidote of magnesium toxicity is 10ml of 10% calcium gluconate –slow IV Restart the magnesium sulphate if urine output improve**

**Management of sever preeclampsia**

**Admit to labor word**

**Request PET investigation**

**Inform senior pediatrician &anesthesiologist on call**

**Start Magnesium sulphate protocol**

**Inform senior obstetrician on call**

**Start antihypertensive agent**

**Continuous close monitoring 24-48 hrs**

# 43.3 Post Partum Fluid Protocol – Pre Eclampsia

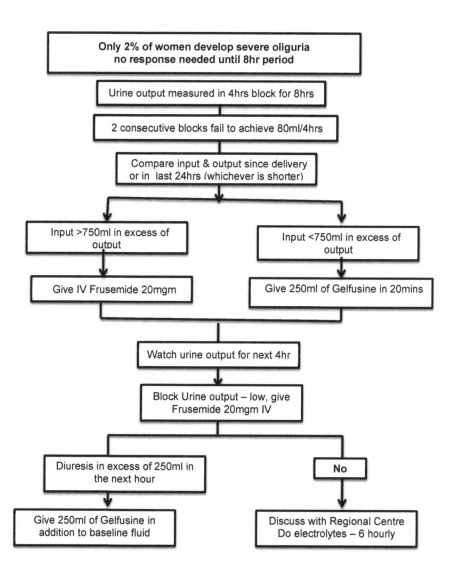

Only 2% of women develop severe oliguria no response needed until 8hr period

Urine output measured in 4hrs block for 8hrs

2 consecutive blocks fail to achieve 80ml/4hrs

Compare input & output since delivery or in last 24hrs (whichever is shorter)

Input >750ml in excess of output

Input <750ml in excess of output

Give IV Frusemide 20mgm

Give 250ml of Gelfusine in 20mins

Watch urine output for next 4hr

Block Urine output – low, give Frusemide 20mgm IV

Diuresis in excess of 250ml in the next hour

No

Give 250ml of Gelfusine in addition to baseline fluid

Discuss with Regional Centre Do electrolytes – 6 hourly

# 43.4   Anti hypertensive

Aim of the therapy is to keep BP<150/80-100mmHg

# 43.5   Choice of antihypertensive

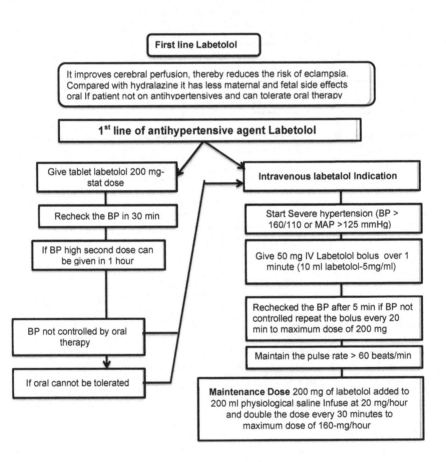

**First line Labetolol**

It improves cerebral perfusion, thereby reduces the risk of eclampsia. Compared with hydralazine it has less maternal and fetal side effects oral If patient not on antihypertensives and can tolerate oral therapy

**1st line of antihypertensive agent Labetolol**

Give tablet labetolol 200 mg-stat dose

Recheck the BP in 30 min

If BP high second dose can be given in 1 hour

BP not controlled by oral therapy

If oral cannot be tolerated

**Intravenous labetalol Indication**

Start Severe hypertension (BP > 160/110 or MAP >125 mmHg)

Give 50 mg IV Labetolol bolus  over 1 minute (10 ml labetolol-5mg/ml)

Rechecked the BP after 5 min if BP not controlled repeat the bolus every 20 min to maximum dose of 200 mg

Maintain the pulse rate > 60 beats/min

**Maintenance Dose** 200 mg of labetolol added to 200 ml physiological saline Infuse at 20 mg/hour and double the dose every 30 minutes to maximum dose of 160-mg/hour

# 43.6  2nd line of antihypertensive agent pathway

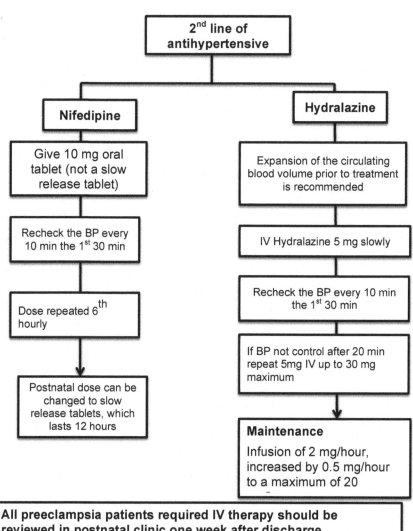

**2nd line of antihypertensive**

**Nifedipine**

Give 10 mg oral tablet (not a slow release tablet)

Recheck the BP every 10 min the 1st 30 min

Dose repeated 6th hourly

Postnatal dose can be changed to slow release tablets, which lasts 12 hours

**Hydralazine**

Expansion of the circulating blood volume prior to treatment is recommended

IV Hydralazine 5 mg slowly

Recheck the BP every 10 min the 1st 30 min

If BP not control after 20 min repeat 5mg IV up to 30 mg maximum

**Maintenance**

Infusion of 2 mg/hour, increased by 0.5 mg/hour to a maximum of 20

**All preeclampsia patients required IV therapy should be reviewed in postnatal clinic one week after discharge**

# 43.7 Seizure prophylaxis Magnesium sulphate protocol

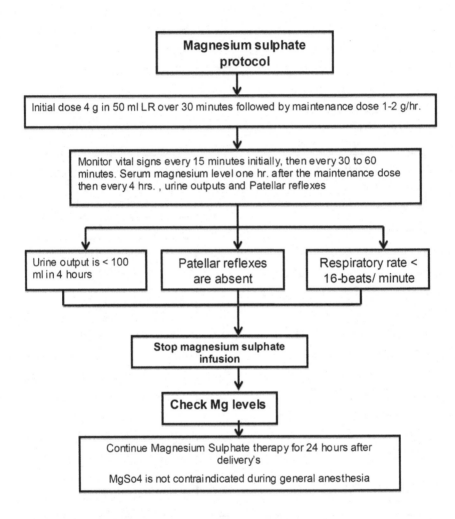

**Magnesium sulphate protocol**

Initial dose 4 g in 50 ml LR over 30 minutes followed by maintenance dose 1-2 g/hr.

Monitor vital signs every 15 minutes initially, then every 30 to 60 minutes. Serum magnesium level one hr. after the maintenance dose then every 4 hrs. , urine outputs and Patellar reflexes

Urine output is < 100 ml in 4 hours

Patellar reflexes are absent

Respiratory rate < 16-beats/ minute

**Stop magnesium sulphate infusion**

**Check Mg levels**

Continue Magnesium Sulphate therapy for 24 hours after delivery's

MgSo4 is not contraindicated during general anesthesia

# 43.8  Treatment Of Magnesium Toxicity

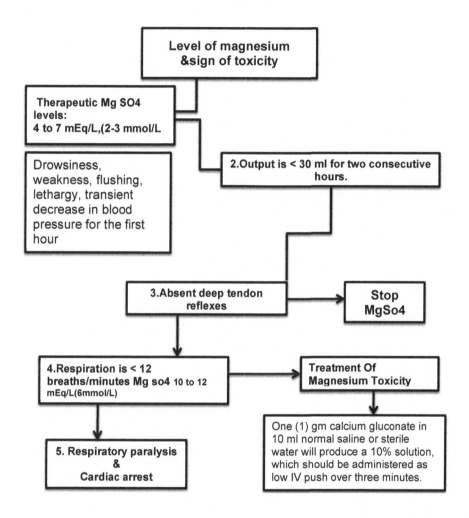

Level of magnesium &sign of toxicity

Therapeutic Mg SO4 levels:
4 to 7 mEq/L,(2-3 mmol/L

Drowsiness, weakness, flushing, lethargy, transient decrease in blood pressure for the first hour

2.Output is < 30 ml for two consecutive hours.

3.Absent deep tendon reflexes

Stop MgSo4

4.Respiration is < 12 breaths/minutes Mg so4 10 to 12 mEq/L(6mmol/L)

Treatment Of Magnesium Toxicity

5. Respiratory paralysis & Cardiac arrest

One (1) gm calcium gluconate in 10 ml normal saline or sterile water will produce a 10% solution, which should be administered as low IV push over three minutes.

# 44  Management of Laboring Women with IDDM/Gestational Diabetes

## 44.1  Time of delivery

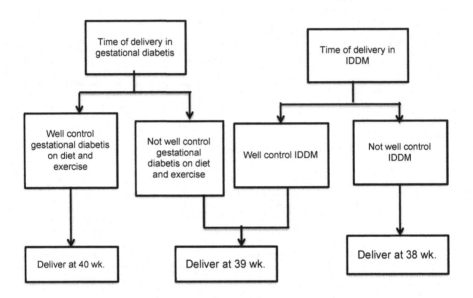

## 44.2   Methods of delivery

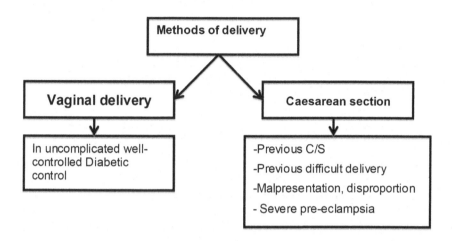

## 44.3   Control of blood glucose during latent phase of labor

Control of blood glucose during latent phase

1.patient is on her usual diet

2.follow SQ insulin protocol

3.Blood glucose monitoring: fasting, 2 hours post prandial

If uncontrolled call the endocrine team (above target or hypoglycemic attack)

# 44.4   Control of blood glucose during during active phase &NPO for elective ceaserian section

Control of blood glucose during during active phase &NPO for elective ceaserian section

1. Start IV insulin infusion+ IV fluid and KCL infusion as in protocol (order by endocrine/internal medicine team)
2. follow serum electrolytes as per protocol.
3. transfer patient to labour ward.
4. follow blood glucose hourly call endocrine /internal medicine team if blood glucose >10mmmol/L or <4 mmol/L
5. inform obstetric &anesthesia registrar.
6. start high-risk monitoring –maternal observations, continuous CTG, maintenance of partogram
7. keep senior obstetrician on call informed about progress. Anticipate shoulder dystocia at birth and follow protocol for shoulder dystocia

# 44.5 Diabetic patient Post delivery pathway

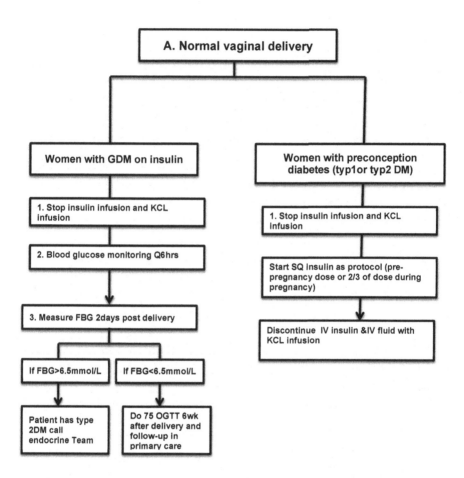

**A. Normal vaginal delivery**

**Women with GDM on insulin**

1. Stop insulin infusion and KCL infusion

2. Blood glucose monitoring Q6hrs

3. Measure FBG 2days post delivery

If FBG>6.5mmol/L

If FBG<6.5mmol/L

Patient has type 2DM call endocrine Team

Do 75 OGTT 6wk after delivery and follow-up in primary care

**Women with preconception diabetes (typ1or typ2 DM)**

1. Stop insulin infusion and KCL infusion

Start SQ insulin as protocol (pre-pregnancy dose or 2/3 of dose during pregnancy)

Discontinue IV insulin &IV fluid with KCL infusion

## 44.6 Diabetic patient on insulin with preterm labor

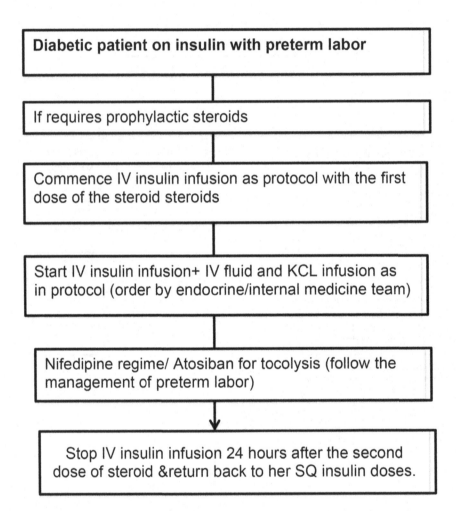

Diabetic patient on insulin with preterm labor

If requires prophylactic steroids

Commence IV insulin infusion as protocol with the first dose of the steroid steroids

Start IV insulin infusion+ IV fluid and KCL infusion as in protocol (order by endocrine/internal medicine team)

Nifedipine regime/ Atosiban for tocolysis (follow the management of preterm labor)

Stop IV insulin infusion 24 hours after the second dose of steroid &return back to her SQ insulin doses.

## 44.7　Diabetic pregnant women with KDA

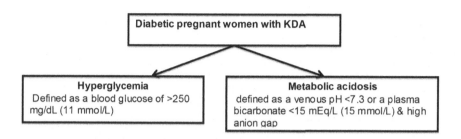

```
Diabetic pregnant women with KDA
```

**Hyperglycemia**
Defined as a blood glucose of >250 mg/dL (11 mmol/L)

**Metabolic acidosis**
defined as a venous pH <7.3 or a plasma bicarbonate <15 mEq/L (15 mmol/L) & high anion gap

## 44.8　Management of DKA

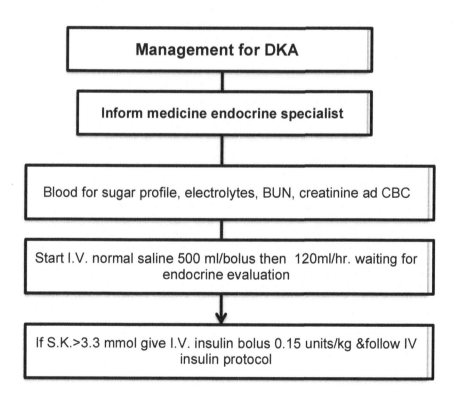

**Management for DKA**

**Inform medicine endocrine specialist**

Blood for sugar profile, electrolytes, BUN, creatinine ad CBC

Start I.V. normal saline 500 ml/bolus then 120ml/hr. waiting for endocrine evaluation

If S.K.>3.3 mmol give I.V. insulin bolus 0.15 units/kg &follow IV insulin protocol

# 45   Antepartum Hemorrhage

## 45.1   Classification of the severity of APH.

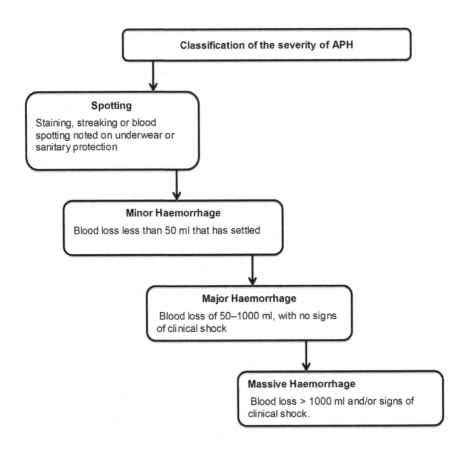

Classification of the severity of APH

**Spotting**

Staining, streaking or blood spotting noted on underwear or sanitary protection

**Minor Haemorrhage**

Blood loss less than 50 ml that has settled

**Major Haemorrhage**

Blood loss of 50–1000 ml, with no signs of clinical shock

**Massive Haemorrhage**

Blood loss > 1000 ml and/or signs of clinical shock.

## 45.2 Causes Antepartum haemorrhage

**Causes Antepartum haemorrhage**

**1.**placental abruption

2.placenta praevia

3.vasa praevia

4.obstetric haemorrhage

5.obstetric hemorrhage

# 45.3 Complications of APH

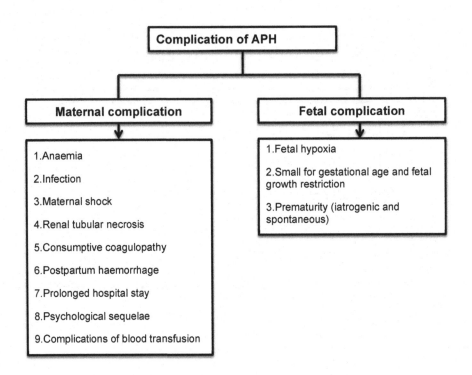

**Complication of APH**

**Maternal complication**

1. Anaemia
2. Infection
3. Maternal shock
4. Renal tubular necrosis
5. Consumptive coagulopathy
6. Postpartum haemorrhage
7. Prolonged hospital stay
8. Psychological sequelae
9. Complications of blood transfusion

**Fetal complication**

1. Fetal hypoxia
2. Small for gestational age and fetal growth restriction
3. Prematurity (iatrogenic and spontaneous)

## 45.4   The main therapeutic goal of management of massive blood loss:

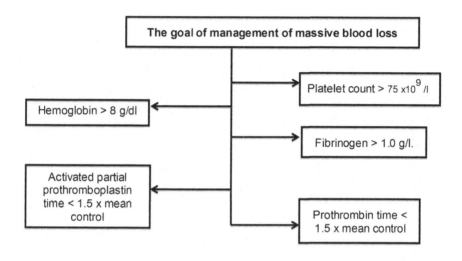

The goal of management of massive blood loss

Platelet count > 75 $\times 10^9$ /l

Hemoglobin > 8 g/dl

Fibrinogen > 1.0 g/l.

Activated partial prothromboplastin time < 1.5 x mean control

Prothrombin time < 1.5 x mean control

# 45.5   Fluid therapy and blood product transfusion

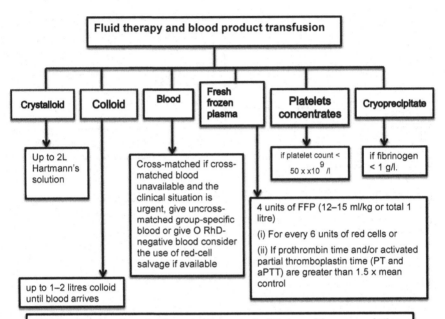

With continuing massive haemorrhage and whilst awaiting coagulation studies, up to 4 units of FFP and 10 units of cryoprecipitate (two packs) may be given empirically.

# 45.6 Antepartum Hemorrhage pathway

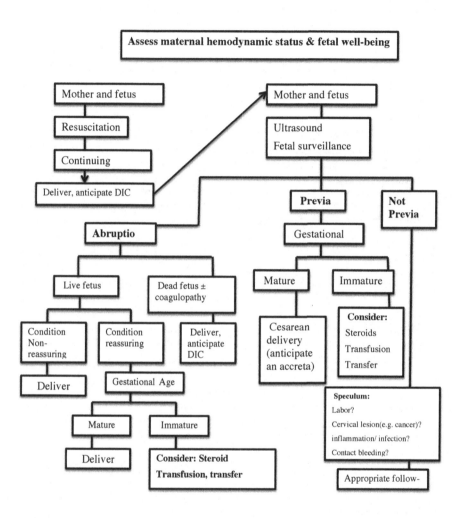

# 46   Genital Herpes during pregnancy

# 46.1   Protocol for Genital Herpes during Labour or <34 weeks gestation

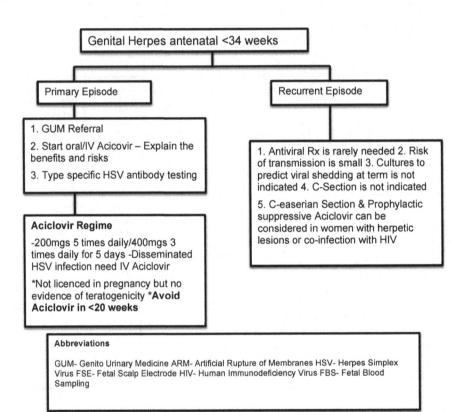

Genital Herpes antenatal <34 weeks

**Primary Episode**

1. GUM Referral

2. Start oral/IV Acicovir – Explain the benefits and risks

3. Type specific HSV antibody testing

**Aciclovir Regime**

-200mgs 5 times daily/400mgs 3 times daily for 5 days -Disseminated HSV infection need IV Aciclovir

*Not licenced in pregnancy but no evidence of teratogenicity *Avoid Aciclovir in <20 weeks**

**Recurrent Episode**

1. Antiviral Rx is rarely needed 2. Risk of transmission is small 3. Cultures to predict viral shedding at term is not indicated 4. C-Section is not indicated

5. C-easerian Section & Prophylactic suppressive Aciclovir can be considered in women with herpetic lesions or co-infection with HIV

**Abbreviations**

GUM- Genito Urinary Medicine ARM- Artificial Rupture of Membranes HSV- Herpes Simplex Virus FSE- Fetal Scalp Electrode HIV- Human Immunodeficiency Virus FBS- Fetal Blood Sampling

# 46.2   Protocol for Genital Herpes during Labour or >34 weeks gestation

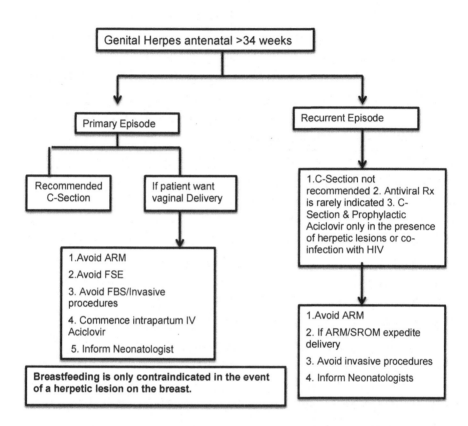

Genital Herpes antenatal >34 weeks

Primary Episode

Recommended C-Section

If patient want vaginal Delivery

1.Avoid ARM

2.Avoid FSE

3. Avoid FBS/Invasive procedures

4. Commence intrapartum IV Aciclovir

5. Inform Neonatologist

**Breastfeeding is only contraindicated in the event of a herpetic lesion on the breast.**

Recurrent Episode

1.C-Section not recommended 2. Antiviral Rx is rarely indicated 3. C-Section & Prophylactic Aciclovir only in the presence of herpetic lesions or co-infection with HIV

1.Avoid ARM

2. If ARM/SROM expedite delivery

3. Avoid invasive procedures

4. Inform Neonatologists

# 47　Instrumental delivery pre-requisites

## 47.1　Pre-requisites for instrumental vaginal delivery

> **Pre-requisites for instrumental vaginal delivery**

Cervix is fully dilated

Fetal head should not be palpable abdominally

Vertex should be at or below spines (0 station) – not caput

Ensure exact position of fetal head

Check mother understands and agrees with the plan.

　Written consent taken for trial in theatre

Ensure analgesia Pudendal block/Epidural/Spinal

Inform Neonatologists to attend delivery

Consultant /Senior (registrar/resident) will decide if instrumental delivery is to be conducted and senior obstetrician should present at the time of conducting instrumental delivery

# 47.2 Instrumental delivery application pathway

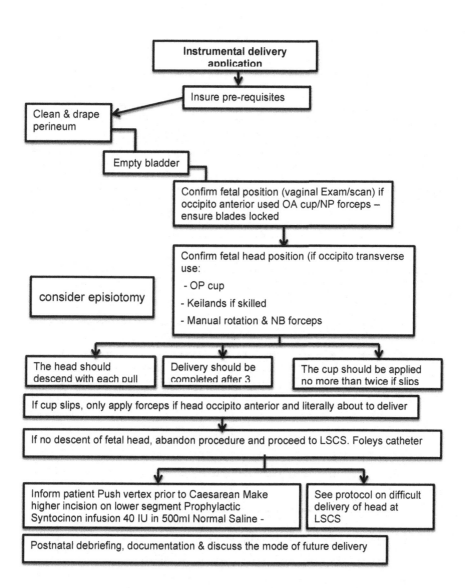

**Instrumental delivery application**

Insure pre-requisites

Clean & drape perineum

Empty bladder

Confirm fetal position (vaginal Exam/scan) if occipito anterior used OA cup/NP forceps – ensure blades locked

Confirm fetal head position (if occipito transverse use:
- OP cup
- Keilands if skilled
- Manual rotation & NB forceps

consider episiotomy

The head should descend with each pull

Delivery should be completed after 3

The cup should be applied no more than twice if slips

If cup slips, only apply forceps if head occipito anterior and literally about to deliver

If no descent of fetal head, abandon procedure and proceed to LSCS. Foleys catheter

Inform patient Push vertex prior to Caesarean Make higher incision on lower segment Prophylactic Syntocinon infusion 40 IU in 500ml Normal Saline -

See protocol on difficult delivery of head at LSCS

Postnatal debriefing, documentation & discuss the mode of future delivery

# 48 Pre Requisites for Caesarean Section guideline

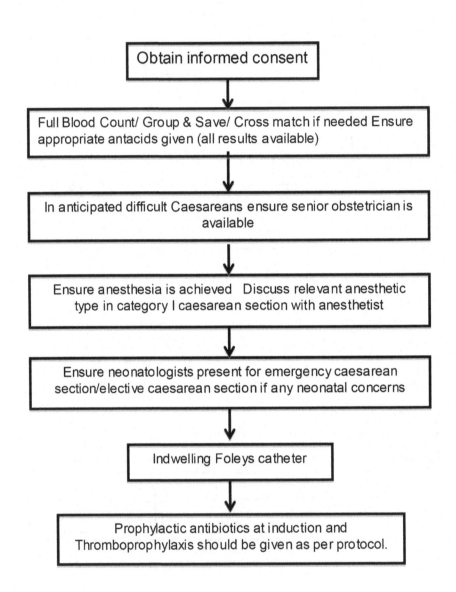

Obtain informed consent

Full Blood Count/ Group & Save/ Cross match if needed Ensure appropriate antacids given (all results available)

In anticipated difficult Caesareans ensure senior obstetrician is available

Ensure anesthesia is achieved   Discuss relevant anesthetic type in category I caesarean section with anesthetist

Ensure neonatologists present for emergency caesarean section/elective caesarean section if any neonatal concerns

Indwelling Foleys catheter

Prophylactic antibiotics at induction and Thromboprophylaxis should be given as per protocol.

# 49   Caesarean Section

# 49.1   Classification Of Caesarean Sections

| Category | Time | Definition |
|----------|------|------------|
| 1A | 30 min | Immediate threat to life of women or fetus, e.g. cord prolapse, uterine rupture, pathological CTG mandate immediate action |
| IB | 30-60 min | Maternal/fetal compromise which is not immediately life-threatening, e.g. APH, failure to progress with maternal or fetal compromise |
| 2 | 1-6hr | No maternal or fetal compromise but needs early delivery (scheduled) e.g. failed IOL or failure to progress |
| 3 | | Delivery timed to suit the woman or staff (elective) |

# 49.2   second Stage Caesarean Section pathway

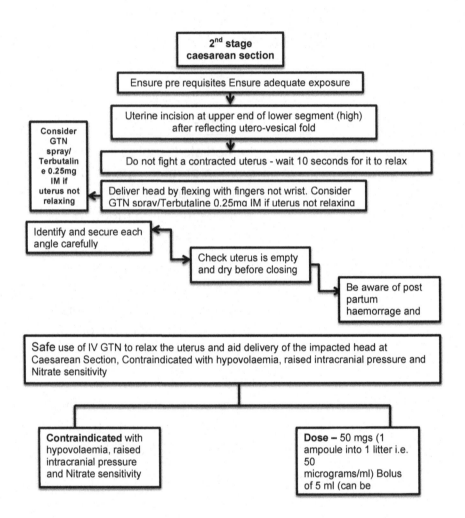

2<sup>nd</sup> stage caesarean section

Ensure pre requisites Ensure adequate exposure

Uterine incision at upper end of lower segment (high) after reflecting utero-vesical fold

Consider GTN spray/ Terbutaline 0.25mg IM if uterus not relaxing

Do not fight a contracted uterus - wait 10 seconds for it to relax

Deliver head by flexing with fingers not wrist. Consider GTN spray/Terbutaline 0.25mg IM if uterus not relaxing

Identify and secure each angle carefully

Check uterus is empty and dry before closing

Be aware of post partum haemorrage and

Safe use of IV GTN to relax the uterus and aid delivery of the impacted head at Caesarean Section, Contraindicated with hypovolaemia, raised intracranial pressure and Nitrate sensitivity

Contraindicated with hypovolaemia, raised intracranial pressure and Nitrate sensitivity

Dose – 50 mgs (1 ampoule into 1 litter i.e. 50 micrograms/ml) Bolus of 5 ml (can be

# 49.3   Prophylactic Antibiotics

Prophylactic Antibiotics

Cefuroxime 1.5g IV on call for Operation Theater

Cefazolin (1 g if ≤60 kg, 2 g for >60 kg) on call for Operation Theater

Ampicillin (2 g)IV  on call for operation theater

**If patient allergic to pencillin**

Metronidazole (500 mg) + gentamicin (1.5 mg/kg) single dose with umbilical cord clamp Or

Clindamycin (600 mg) plus gentamicin (1.5 mg/kg) single dose with umbilical cord clamp

# 50  Breech Delivery

**Breech in labour**

-Council the patient regarding the mode of delivery by the senior registrar
-Confirm the presentation by ultrasound
-Delivery should be conducted by expert regestrsr, senior registrar
- An Anaesthetist and Paediatrician should be present at the delivery.
-Discuss the use of syntocinon if needed with consultant

# 50.1 Management of Breech Presentation in laboring pathway (Expected and Unexpected Breech)

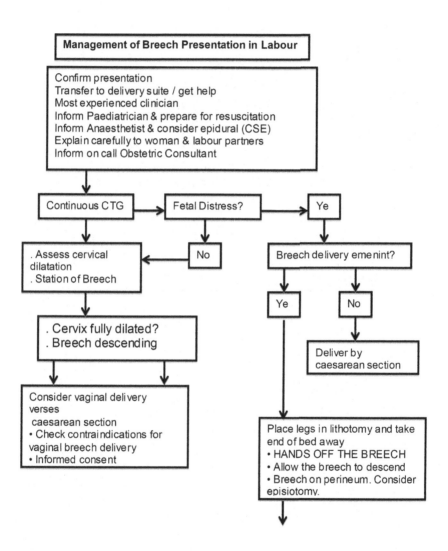

**Management of Breech Presentation in Labour**

Confirm presentation
Transfer to delivery suite / get help
Most experienced clinician
Inform Paediatrician & prepare for resuscitation
Inform Anaesthetist & consider epidural (CSE)
Explain carefully to woman & labour partners
Inform on call Obstetric Consultant

Continuous CTG → Fetal Distress? → Ye

No

. Assess cervical dilatation
. Station of Breech

Breech delivery emenint?

Ye            No

Deliver by caesarean section

. Cervix fully dilated?
. Breech descending

Consider vaginal delivery verses
caesarean section
• Check contraindications for vaginal breech delivery
• Informed consent

Place legs in lithotomy and take end of bed away
• HANDS OFF THE BREECH
• Allow the breech to descend
• Breech on perineum. Consider episiotomy.

Place legs in lithotomy and take end of bed away
• HANDS OFF THE BREECH
• Allow the breech to descend
• Breech on perineum. Consider episiotomy.

Place legs in lithotomy and take end of bed away
• HANDS OFF THE BREECH
• Allow the breech to descend
• Breech on perineum. Consider episiotomy.

With further descent, legs usually deliver without handling.
• If delay with extended legs, deliver by flexion at knee joint and extension at hips
• DO NOT ALLOW BABY'S BACK TO ROTATE POSTERIORLY
• BABY'S SACRUM MUST BE UPPERMOST IF WOMAN IS SUPINE
• Allow arms to deliver.
• If arms extended and delaying progress, LOVSETT'S manoeuvre
• Allow breech and head to descend until the nape of the neck is visible

Mauriceau-Smellie Veit manoeuvre Breech Trouble Shooting.
• Forceps, if required, by skilled obstetrician

# 50.2 Complecated breech delivery pathway

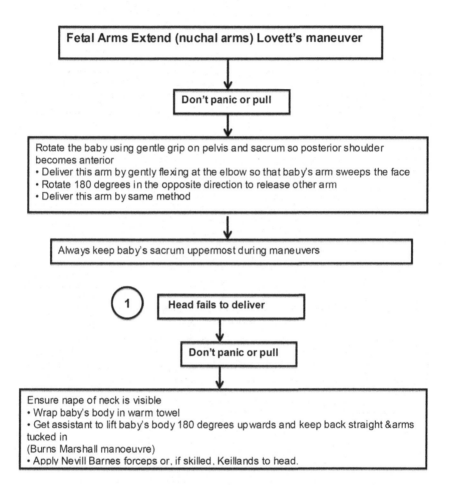

Fetal Arms Extend (nuchal arms) Lovett's maneuver

Don't panic or pull

Rotate the baby using gentle grip on pelvis and sacrum so posterior shoulder becomes anterior
• Deliver this arm by gently flexing at the elbow so that baby's arm sweeps the face
• Rotate 180 degrees in the opposite direction to release other arm
• Deliver this arm by same method

Always keep baby's sacrum uppermost during maneuvers

1  Head fails to deliver

Don't panic or pull

Ensure nape of neck is visible
• Wrap baby's body in warm towel
• Get assistant to lift baby's body 180 degrees upwards and keep back straight & arms tucked in
(Burns Marshall manoeuvre)
• Apply Nevill Barnes forceps or, if skilled, Keillands to head.

# 51   Twin Delivery

## 51.1   Twin management pathway

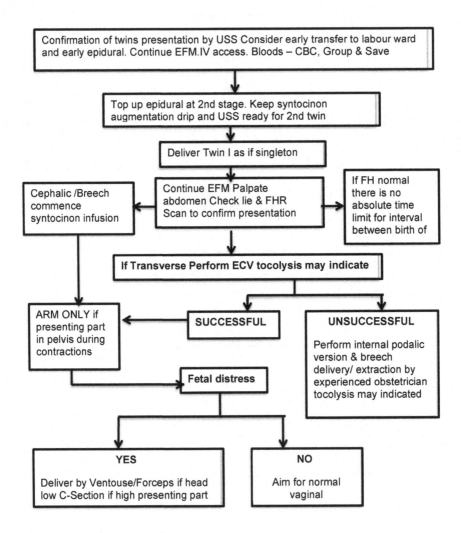

Confirmation of twins presentation by USS Consider early transfer to labour ward and early epidural. Continue EFM.IV access. Bloods – CBC, Group & Save

Top up epidural at 2nd stage. Keep syntocinon augmentation drip and USS ready for 2nd twin

Deliver Twin I as if singleton

Cephalic /Breech commence syntocinon infusion

Continue EFM Palpate abdomen Check lie & FHR Scan to confirm presentation

If FH normal there is no absolute time limit for interval between birth of

If Transverse Perform ECV tocolysis may indicate

ARM ONLY if presenting part in pelvis during contractions

SUCCESSFUL

UNSUCCESSFUL

Perform internal podalic version & breech delivery/ extraction by experienced obstetrician tocolysis may indicated

Fetal distress

YES

Deliver by Ventouse/Forceps if head low C-Section if high presenting part

NO

Aim for normal vaginal

## 51.2 Twin delivery Management pathway

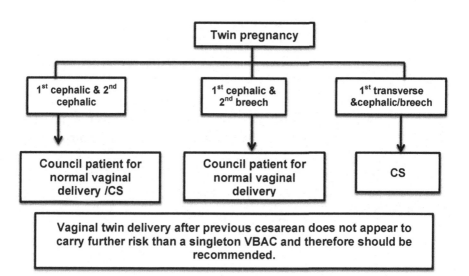

| Twin pregnancy | | |
|---|---|---|
| 1st cephalic & 2nd cephalic | 1st cephalic & 2nd breech | 1st transverse &cephalic/breech |
| Council patient for normal vaginal delivery /CS | Council patient for normal vaginal delivery | CS |

Vaginal twin delivery after previous cesarean does not appear to carry further risk than a singleton VBAC and therefore should be recommended.

# 51.3 Analgesia

Analgesia

## 1.1 Maternal choice is of key importance and all options be considered. Epidural is the method of choice.

-The benefit of effective epidural it allows rapid top-up for a trial of instrumental delivery, external or internal version of the second twin or CS if there are problems.

-The anesthetist should be aware of the progress of labour
-Elective epidural top-up for the delivery of the second twin will facilitate manipulation, instrumental delivery and rapid top-up for CS.

# 52 Shoulder Dystocia management pathway

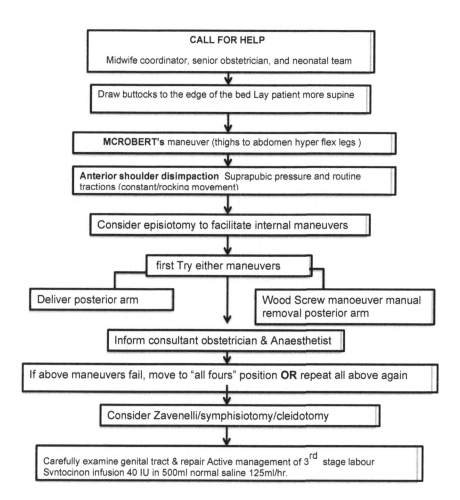

CALL FOR HELP

Midwife coordinator, senior obstetrician, and neonatal team

Draw buttocks to the edge of the bed Lay patient more supine

MCROBERT's maneuver (thighs to abdomen hyper flex legs )

Anterior shoulder disimpaction  Suprapubic pressure and routine tractions (constant/rocking movement)

Consider episiotomy to facilitate internal maneuvers

first Try either maneuvers

Deliver posterior arm

Wood Screw manoeuver manual removal posterior arm

Inform consultant obstetrician & Anaesthetist

If above maneuvers fail, move to "all fours" position OR repeat all above again

Consider Zavenelli/symphisiotomy/cleidotomy

Carefully examine genital tract & repair Active management of $3^{rd}$ stage labour Syntocinon infusion 40 IU in 500ml normal saline 125ml/hr.

# 53 Management of Cord Prolapse

# 53.1 Definitions Cord Presentation

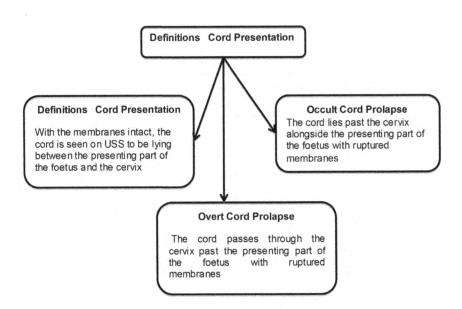

**Definitions Cord Presentation**

**Definitions Cord Presentation**

With the membranes intact, the cord is seen on USS to be lying between the presenting part of the foetus and the cervix

**Occult Cord Prolapse**
The cord lies past the cervix alongside the presenting part of the foetus with ruptured membranes

**Overt Cord Prolapse**

The cord passes through the cervix past the presenting part of the foetus with ruptured membranes

# 53.2   Cord prolapse management pathway

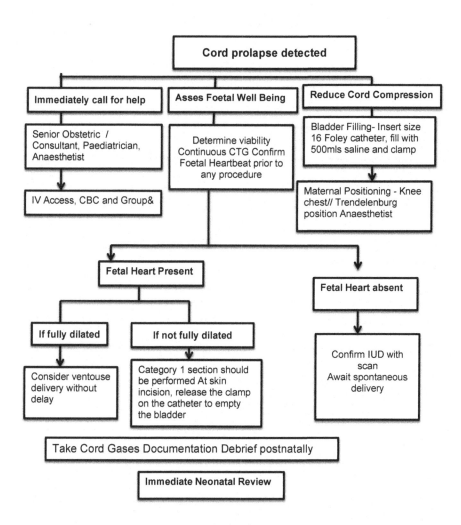

Cord prolapse detected

**Immediately call for help**

Senior Obstetric / Consultant, Paediatrician, Anaesthetist

IV Access, CBC and Group&

**Asses Foetal Well Being**

Determine viability Continuous CTG Confirm Foetal Heartbeat prior to any procedure

**Reduce Cord Compression**

Bladder Filling- Insert size 16 Foley catheter, fill with 500mls saline and clamp

Maternal Positioning - Knee chest// Trendelenburg position Anaesthetist

**Fetal Heart Present**

**If fully dilated**

Consider ventouse delivery without delay

**If not fully dilated**

Category 1 section should be performed At skin incision, release the clamp on the catheter to empty the bladder

**Fetal Heart absent**

Confirm IUD with scan Await spontaneous delivery

Take Cord Gases Documentation Debrief postnatally

**Immediate Neonatal Review**

# 54   Uterine Inversion

## 54.1   Suspect uterine inversion

Suspect  uterine inversion

**Recognition**

- Severe lower abdominal pain in 3rd Stage of labour
- Haemorrhage (94%)
- Shock that is out of proportion to blood loss owing to vagal stimulation
- Placenta may or may not be in place
- uterine fundus not palpable per abdomen
- Pelvic examination shows mass in the vagina or outside the introitus

# 54.2   Management of uterine inversion

```
┌─────────────────────────────────────────┐
│     Management of uterine inversion      │
└─────────────────────────────────────────┘

┌─────────────────────────────────────────────────────────────┐
│ Call for help from experienced obstetrician/ Anaesthetist/   │
│ midwives                                                     │
└─────────────────────────────────────────────────────────────┘

┌─────────────────────────────────┐
│    Stop Syntocinon if on flow   │
└─────────────────────────────────┘
```

┌───────────────────────────────────────────────────────────────────┐
│ **Take the anti shock measures**                                  │
│                                                                   │
│ • Insert 2 wide bore cannula (14 to 16G)                          │
│                                                                   │
│ • Collect blood for FBC, coagulation studies, group and cross     │
│   match 4 -6 units                                                │
│                                                                   │
│ • Start fluid replacements immediately (crystalloids)             │
│                                                                   │
│ • Monitor BP, pulse, urine output, O2 saturation continuously     │
└───────────────────────────────────────────────────────────────────┘

```
              ┌─────────────────────────┐
              │   Transfer to theatre   │
              └─────────────────────────┘
```

┌───────────────────────────────────────────────────────────────────┐
│ **After given appropriate analgesia**                             │
│                                                                   │
│ Consider tocolytics to facilitate replacement of uterus (MgSO4    │
│ 2-4g IV 5 mints)Terbutaline 0.25 mgm IV/Nitroglycerine 100 mgm IV │
│                                                                   │
│ Attempt to reposition the uterus                                  │
│                                                                   │
│ -Manual replacement (Johnson maneuver)                            │
│                                                                   │
│ -O'Sullivan's technique infuse 2-3 liters warm saline into        │
│ posterior fornix of the vagina (use Ventouse silicon cup)         │
│                                                                   │
│ -Surgery - *Huntingdon's method **Houltains technique             │
└───────────────────────────────────────────────────────────────────┘

┌───────────────────────────────────────────────────────────────────┐
│ -Oxytocin administered after repositioning (post replacement)/    │
│ -Do not remove placenta, leave until after repositioning / IV     │
│ prophylactic antibiotics /-Thromboprophylaxis as per protocol     │
└───────────────────────────────────────────────────────────────────┘

# 55   Ruptured uterus

# 55.1   Risk factors for uterine rupture

**Risk factor**

Obesity
• uterine scar
• Oxytocic in the multigravida woman or with previous caesarean scar
• Gran multiparty
• Diagnosed CPD
• Malpresentation
• Placenta accrete
• Macrosomic

**Warning sign**

Scar pain and tenderness
• Persistent pain between contractions
• Vaginal bleeding
• Fetal distress
• Fetal heart rate decelerati fetus
• Uterine abnormality
• Prior

# 55.2 Ruptured uterus management pathway

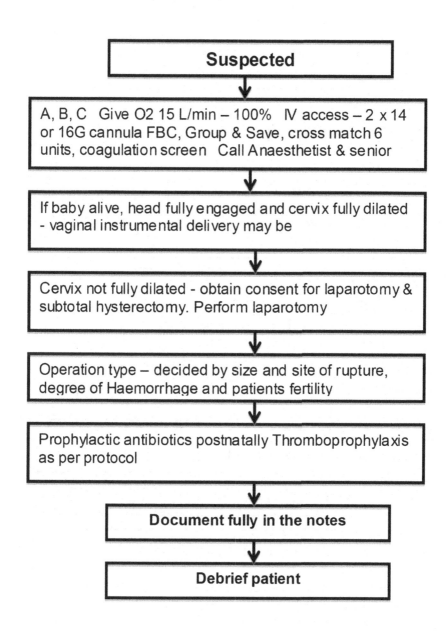

**Suspected**

A, B, C  Give O2 15 L/min – 100%  IV access – 2 x 14 or 16G cannula FBC, Group & Save, cross match 6 units, coagulation screen  Call Anaesthetist & senior

If baby alive, head fully engaged and cervix fully dilated - vaginal instrumental delivery may be

Cervix not fully dilated - obtain consent for laparotomy & subtotal hysterectomy. Perform laparotomy

Operation type – decided by size and site of rupture, degree of Haemorrhage and patients fertility

Prophylactic antibiotics postnatally Thromboprophylaxis as per protocol

**Document fully in the notes**

**Debrief patient**

# 56   Retained Placenta

## 56.1   Definition

Definition: Placenta undelivered after 30mins

## 56.2   Retained placenta management

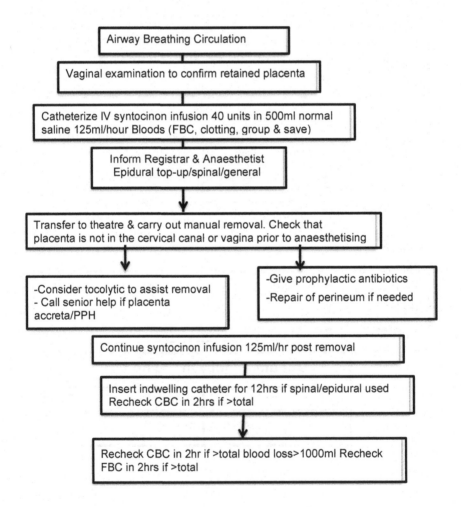

Airway Breathing Circulation

Vaginal examination to confirm retained placenta

Catheterize IV syntocinon infusion 40 units in 500ml normal saline 125ml/hour Bloods (FBC, clotting, group & save)

Inform Registrar & Anaesthetist
Epidural top-up/spinal/general

Transfer to theatre & carry out manual removal. Check that placenta is not in the cervical canal or vagina prior to anaesthetising

-Consider tocolytic to assist removal
- Call senior help if placenta accreta/PPH

-Give prophylactic antibiotics
-Repair of perineum if needed

Continue syntocinon infusion 125ml/hr post removal

Insert indwelling catheter for 12hrs if spinal/epidural used
Recheck CBC in 2hrs if >total

Recheck CBC in 2hr if >total blood loss>1000ml Recheck FBC in 2hrs if >total

## 57 Care plan for women in labor if blood not available

IV access.

CBC, Group & Save.

Inform consultant obstetrician and Anaesthetist.

Active management of 3$^{rd}$ stage of labor.

Do not leave the patient alone for first hour after delivery.

IV Oxytocin infusion if any risk factors of PPH present.

## 57.1 Management Of Postpartum Anaemia

1.Severe anemia – involve hematologist. Give oxygen use recombinant   human erythropoietin's 300 units/kg – three-weekly subcutaneously.

Augment with iron, vitamin B12 and folic acid.

2.IV Ferrous inject 1 gram if patient > 70 Kg- 15 minute infusion.

3.Consider elective ventilation in ICU.

4.Hyperbaric oxygen therapy – in life threatening anemia.
Contacts:  Hospital Liaison Committee for Jehovah's Witnesses

## 57.2 Management in active hemorrhage in labor if blood not avialable

## 57.3 1st step in active hemorrhage management

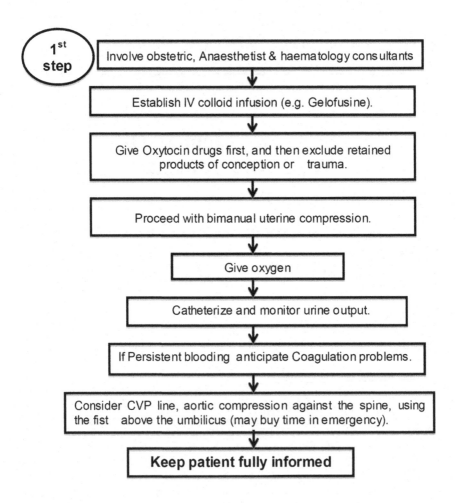

**1st step** → Involve obstetric, Anaesthetist & haematology consultants

Establish IV colloid infusion (e.g. Gelofusine).

Give Oxytocin drugs first, and then exclude retained products of conception or trauma.

Proceed with bimanual uterine compression.

Give oxygen

Catheterize and monitor urine output.

If Persistent blooding anticipate Coagulation problems.

Consider CVP line, aortic compression against the spine, using the fist above the umbilicus (may buy time in emergency).

**Keep patient fully informed**

## 57.4 2nd step in active hemorrhage management pathway

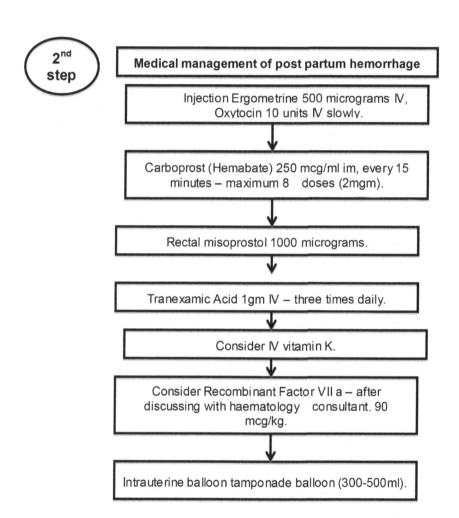

**2<sup>nd</sup> step**

**Medical management of post partum hemorrhage**

Injection Ergometrine 500 micrograms IV, Oxytocin 10 units IV slowly.

Carboprost (Hemabate) 250 mcg/ml im, every 15 minutes – maximum 8 doses (2mgm).

Rectal misoprostol 1000 micrograms.

Tranexamic Acid 1gm IV – three times daily.

Consider IV vitamin K.

Consider Recombinant Factor VII a – after discussing with haematology consultant. 90 mcg/kg.

Intrauterine balloon tamponade balloon (300-500ml).

# 57.5 Surgical management of post partum hemorrhage pathway

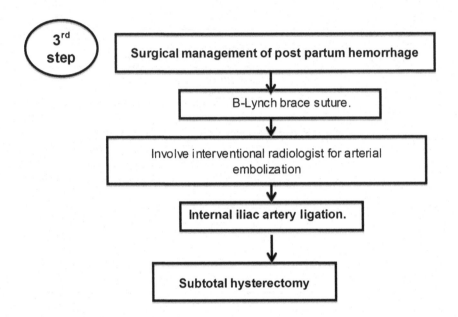

# 58 Management of Post Partum Hemorrhage

## 58.1 Risk Factors for Post Partum Hemorrhage

Risk Factors for Post Partum Hemorrhage

**Presenting antenatally and associated with a substantial increase in the incidence of PPH**

-Suspected or proven placental abruption Thrombin

-Known placenta previa Tone

-Multiple pregnancies Tone

-Pre-eclampsia/gestational hypertension

**Presenting antenatally and associated with a significant increase in the incidence of PPH**

Previous PPH
Asian ethnicity
Obesity (BMI >35) G Anemia (<9 g/dl)

**Becoming apparent during labour and delivery; these factors should prompt extra vigilance among clinical staff**

-Delivery by elective CS

- Retained placenta

-Operative vaginal delivery

- Big baby (> 4 kg)

-Age (>40 years, not multiparous)

- Induction of labour

- Mediolateral episiotomy

-Prolonged labour (> 12 hrs)

-Pyrexia in labour

-Delivery by emergency CS

# 58.2   Definition& general measure to stabilize patient with PPH pathway

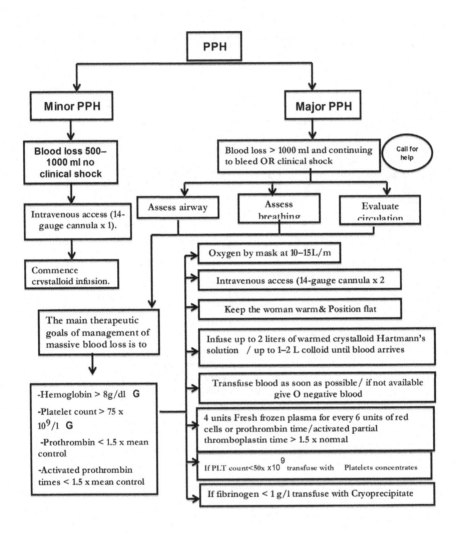

# 59   Massive transfusion

## 59.1   Management of patient with massive blood loss

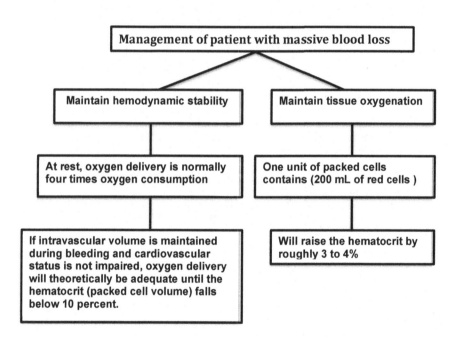

Massive transfusion, defined as
The replacement by transfusion of more than 50 percent of a patient's blood volume in 12 to 24 hours,

Management of patient with massive blood loss

Maintain hemodynamic stability

Maintain tissue oxygenation

At rest, oxygen delivery is normally four times oxygen consumption

One unit of packed cells contains (200 mL of red cells )

If intravascular volume is maintained during bleeding and cardiovascular status is not impaired, oxygen delivery will theoretically be adequate until the hematocrit (packed cell volume) falls below 10 percent.

Will raise the hematocrit by roughly 3 to 4%

# 59.2   Treatment of patient with severe hypovolemia or hypovolemic shock

```
┌─────────────────────────────────────────────────────────────────┐
│ Treatment of patient with severe hypovolemia or hypovolemic shock │
└─────────────────────────────────────────────────────────────────┘
                    ┌──────────────────────────────┐
                    │ The principle of fluid resuscitation │
                    └──────────────────────────────┘
```

**The rate of fluid replacement**

**The type of fluid infused**

2-3 liters of isotonic saline are initially given as rapidly as possible in an attempt to restore tissue perfusion

Fluid repletion should continue at the initial rapid rate as long as the systemic blood pressure remains low. Clinical signs, including blood pressure, urine output, mental status, and peripheral perfusion, are often adequate to guide resuscitation.

A central venous catheter should be considered in patients who fail to respond to initial fluid resuscitation

**The role for buffer therapy in patients with concurrent lactic acidosis**

**Saline solutions are equally effective as colloid in expanding the plasma volume** Colloid-containing solutions are not more effective in preserving pulmonary function

Starch solutions have been associated with coagulopathy, and increased risk of acute kidney injury

**Lactated-Ringers** solution or 0.45% saline solution with 75 mmol/L of sodium bicarbonate ) be used instead of isotonic saline for large volume resuscitation.

Large volume resuscitation using isotonic saline may be associated with hyperchloremic metabolic acidosis &renal vasoconstriction and decreased glomerular filtration further disturbed electrolyte in ICU patient

Patients with marked hypo perfusion may develop lactic acidosis, leading to a reduction in extracellular pH below 7.10. Sodium bicarbonate has been added to the replacement fluid in this setting

# 59.3 Complication of massive blood transfusion

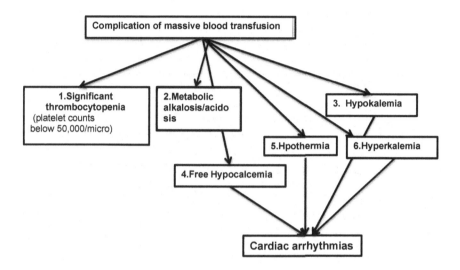

Complication of massive blood transfusion

1.Significant thrombocytopenia (platelet counts below 50,000/micro)

2.Metabolic alkalosis/acidosis

3. Hypokalemia

5.Hpothermia

6.Hyperkalemia

4.Free Hypocalcemia

Cardiac arrhythmias

# 59.4   If the Patient require blood transfusion>5 unit

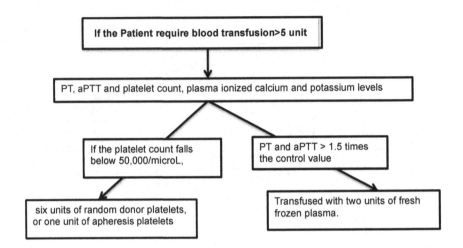

If the Patient require blood transfusion>5 unit

PT, aPTT and platelet count, plasma ionized calcium and potassium levels

If the platelet count falls below 50,000/microL,

PT and aPTT > 1.5 times the control value

six units of random donor platelets, or one unit of apheresis platelets

Transfused with two units of fresh frozen plasma.

# 59.5 Complication of massive blood transfusion

Complication of massive blood transfusion

**1.Significant thrombocytopenia**
(platelet counts below 50,000/micro)

For each 10 to 12 units of transfused red cells can produce a 50 percent fall in the platelet count

**One apheresis concentrate should increase the platelet count by 5000 to 10,000/microL**

**2.Metabolic alkalosis/acidosis**

The pH of a unit of blood at the time of collection is 7.10 The pH then falls 0.1 pH unit/week due to the production of lactic and pyruvic acids by the red cells.

Citrate will generate a total of 23 meq of bicarbonate in each unit of blood

Maintain: Oxygenation, Cardiac output &Tissue perfusion

Metabolic alkalosis can occur if the renal ischemia or underlying renal disease prevents the excess bicarbonate from being excreted in the urine. This may be accompanied by hypokalemia as potassium moves into cells in exchange for hydrogen ions that move out of the cells to minimize the degree of extracellular alkalosis

**3.Hypokalemia**

Blood is anticoagulated with sodium citrate which increase the bicarbonate and this lead to metabolic alkalosis H+ shift from intracellular to extracellular ,k will shift to intracellular causing hypokalemia

## 4. Hypocalcemia

Citrate will combine with ionized calcium this will lead to significant fall in the plasma free calcium concentration and increase in Free hypocalcemia which lead to Paresthesias & cardiac arrhythmias treat hypocalcemia by10 %calcium gluconate give 10 to 20ml for every 500 mL of blood infused.

## 5.Hpothermia

Use fluid warmers, Remove wet linen, Provide warmer blankets and monitor temperature at least Q 15 minutes

## 6. Hyperkalemia

Patient with renal impairment may develop hyperkalemia because of potassium leakage due to prolonged blood storage or irradiation

**To minimize the risk of hyperkalemia**

1.Select only red cells collected less than five days prior to transfusion.2.Any unit of red cells can be washed immediately before infusion to remove extracellular potassium

Patients with severe massive blood replacement, and coagulopathy have improved survival when the ratio of transfused FFP (units) to transfused platelets (units) to red cells (units) approaches **1:1:1**

## Laboratory

### Base line investigation

CBC, coagulation profile (PT, APTT, fibrinogen), biochemistry (electrolytes and liver function tests, include Ca2+ and lactate), arterial blood gases (ABG)

### Follow up investigation

CBC, coagulation profile (PT, APTT, fibrinogen), serum electrolytes include Ca2+ and lactate, (ABG)

### Target Results

-pH greater than 7.20

-Base deficit greater than minus 6

-Lactate less than 4 mmol/L

-Ca2+ greater than 1.1 mmol/L

Platelets greater than $50 \times 10^9$/L

-PT and aPTT less than 1.5 x normal

-Fibrinogen greater than 2.5 g/L

## 59.6   Causes for PPH 'the four Ts'

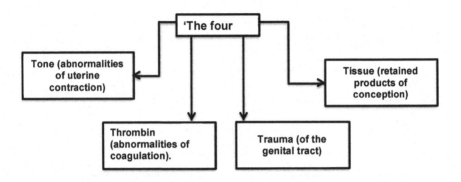

'The four

Tone (abnormalities of uterine contraction)

Tissue (retained products of conception)

Thrombin (abnormalities of coagulation).

Trauma (of the genital tract)

# 59.7 Medical Management of uterine atony pathway

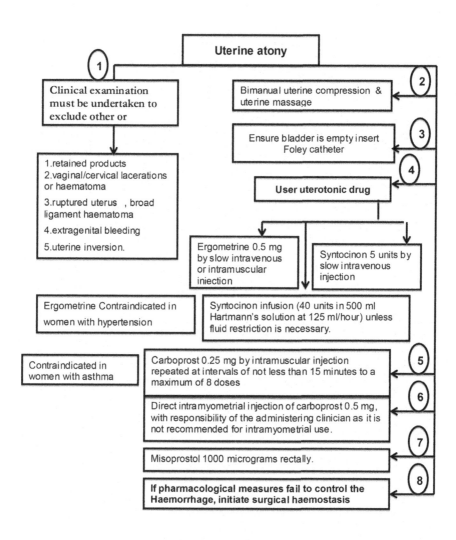

**Uterine atony**

**1** Clinical examination must be undertaken to exclude other or

1. retained products
2. vaginal/cervical lacerations or haematoma
3. ruptured uterus , broad ligament haematoma
4. extragenital bleeding
5. uterine inversion.

**2** Bimanual uterine compression & uterine massage

**3** Ensure bladder is empty insert Foley catheter

**4** **User uterotonic drug**

Ergometrine 0.5 mg by slow intravenous or intramuscular injection

Syntocinon 5 units by slow intravenous injection

Ergometrine Contraindicated in women with hypertension

Syntocinon infusion (40 units in 500 ml Hartmann's solution at 125 ml/hour) unless fluid restriction is necessary.

Contraindicated in women with asthma

**5** Carboprost 0.25 mg by intramuscular injection repeated at intervals of not less than 15 minutes to a maximum of 8 doses

**6** Direct intramyometrial injection of carboprost 0.5 mg, with responsibility of the administering clinician as it is not recommended for intramyometrial use.

**7** Misoprostol 1000 micrograms rectally.

**8** If pharmacological measures fail to control the Haemorrhage, initiate surgical haemostasis

# 59.8 Surgical management of uterine atony pathway

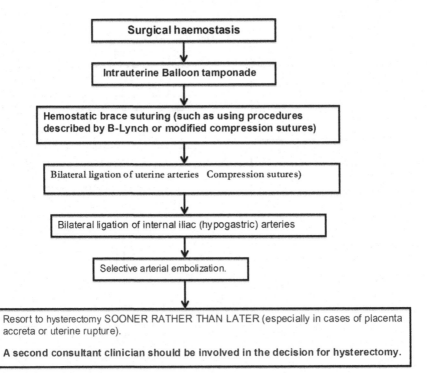

Surgical haemostasis

↓

Intrauterine Balloon tamponade

↓

Hemostatic brace suturing (such as using procedures described by B-Lynch or modified compression sutures)

↓

Bilateral ligation of uterine arteries   Compression sutures)

↓

Bilateral ligation of internal iliac (hypogastric) arteries

↓

Selective arterial embolization.

↓

Resort to hysterectomy SOONER RATHER THAN LATER (especially in cases of placenta accreta or uterine rupture).

**A second consultant clinician should be involved in the decision for hysterectomy.**

# 60    Intra-Partum Collapse

## 60.1    Uterine Rupture

> **Uterine Rupture**

> Note any previous history of uterine surgery, e.g.
> caesarean section, myomectomy, ectopic pregnancy

## 60.2    Eclampsia

> Eclampsia

> The women may be admitted from home fitted
> with no previous history of PIH.

# 60.3   Pulmonary Embolism Amniotic Fluid Embolism

Pulmonary Embolism Amniotic Fluid Embolism

**Presentation of Amniotic Fluid Embolism**
-Sudden dyspnea, hypoxia and hypotension, which may be followed in minutes by cardio-respiratory arrest.
- Grand mal seizures.
-In survival left ventricular failure may develop in clinical picture consistent with adult respiratory distress

**Risk factors for amniotic embolus include**

•High parity.
•Excessive or strong contractions.
•The use of oxytocin drugs, in particular a single Intravenous bolus dose of Syntocinon or Syntometrine.
•Over distension of the uterus, e.g. Polyhydramnios.
•Uterine rupture.
The diagnosis can only be confirmed after the event by finding evidence of fetal squamous cells and much in peripheral vasculature.
Blood should be taken during the acute event for this purpose especially if a Swan Ganz catheter is inserted.

## 60.4   Neurological Causes

**Neurological Causes**

Epilepsy
Intracranial haemorrhage
Cerebral infarction.

## 60.5   Cardiac causes.

Cardiac causes.

Known case of cardiac disease ,patient seen & evaluated by cardiologist

Condition that occure suddenly in labour room causing intrapartum colaps arrhythmia or myocardial infarction due to ischemic heart disease can present in pregnancy as can cardiomyopathy and rupture aortic aneurysm.

A chest X-ray and ECG should be considered in any women presenting with chest pain particularly is she has hypertension

# 60.6   Cardiac Arrest

Cardiac arrest is the failure of the heart to pump sufficient blood to keep the brain alive. Circulatory arrest-complete or virtual complete cessation of blood of blood to the vital organs.

## Aim Of Cardio Pulmonary Resuscitation

### 1.To restore oxygenated to the brain.

1•External cardiac massages.
2•Ventilation with proper oxygenation.
3• Compression to ventilation ratio 5:1 with two resuscitators. If pulse is palpable stop cardiac massage and observe for 5 seconds, to see if spontaneous breathing and pulse have been restored.
Call cardiologist and ICU team.

### 2.To restore adequate cardiac output.

1. Return of femoral pulse.
2. Reliable blood pressure monitoring.
**IN THE PRESENCE OF RELATIVELY NORMAL ECG**

### 3.To manage the patient following the resuscitation.

Done by cardiology team

# 61 Management of delivery in cardiac disease patient

# 61.1 Aim and purpose

Aim and purpose

Timing and mode of delivery should be discussed in advance in a multidisciplinary team consisting of at least an obstetrician, an anesthesiologist, and a cardiologist.

The patient's should be thoroughly counseled about the delivery plan and potential complications.

A written record should be available at all times for all involved caregivers and should include plans to manage foreseeable complications.

# 61.2   Timing of delivery

| Timing of delivery |
|---|

| Asymptomatic women in good condition | Wait for spontaneous labor |
|---|---|
| In women with complex lesions<br><br>- Severe cardiac dysfunction<br>- Heart failure<br>- Aortic dilatation<br>- Eisenmenger syndrome<br>- Mechanical valve switched to heparin | Planned delivery might be more appropriate.<br><br>Maternal or fetal condition might warrant a planned delivery before 37 weeks |

# 61.3  Mode of delivery

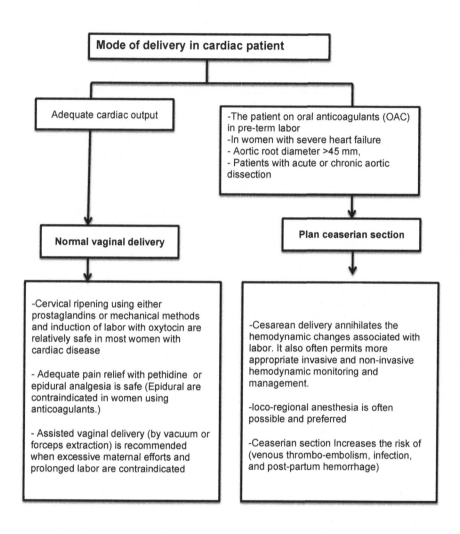

Mode of delivery in cardiac patient

Adequate cardiac output

-The patient on oral anticoagulants (OAC) in pre-term labor
-In women with severe heart failure
- Aortic root diameter >45 mm,
- Patients with acute or chronic aortic dissection

Normal vaginal delivery

Plan ceaserian section

-Cervical ripening using either prostaglandins or mechanical methods and induction of labor with oxytocin are relatively safe in most women with cardiac disease

- Adequate pain relief with pethidine  or epidural analgesia is safe (Epidural are contraindicated in women using anticoagulants.)

- Assisted vaginal delivery (by vacuum or forceps extraction) is recommended when excessive maternal efforts and prolonged labor are contraindicated

-Cesarean delivery annihilates the hemodynamic changes associated with labor. It also often permits more appropriate invasive and non-invasive hemodynamic monitoring and management.

-loco-regional anesthesia is often possible and preferred

-Ceaserian section Increases the risk of (venous thrombo-embolism, infection, and post-partum hemorrhage)

# 61.4   Prophylaxis antibiotics in cardiac patient

Prophylaxis antibiotics in cardiac patient

Preventive antibiotics are generally recommended for high risk patient with the following conditions

1.A prosthetic heart valve

2.Valve repair with prosthetic material

3.A prior history of Infected Endocarditis

4.Many congenital (from birth) heart abnormalities, such as single ventricle states, transposition of the great arteries, and tetralogy of Fallot, even if the abnormality has been repaired. Patent foramen ovale,

5. Pregnant women who are at highest risk for Infected Endocarditis should take an antibiotic before certain dental, oral, or upper respiratory tract procedures

A pregnant woman who has a high risk of Infected Endocarditis does NOT usually need antibiotic prophylaxis before a normal vaginal delivery or cesarean section. Antibiotics may be recommended before labor or cesarean section for other reasons, including prevention of complications related to group B Streptococcus.

# 61.5 Post-partum period in cardiac patient

**Post-partum period in cardiac patient**

-Manage the 3rd stage of labour by oxytocin intravenous infusion
-Intravenous bolus of oxytocine might cause a sudden fall in cardiac output
- Intravenous prostaglandins, can cause coronary vasospasms

**Post-partum period in cardiac patient**

**High-risk patients**

**Low -risk patients**

**(Patients with diminished left ventricular function)Consider**

-Several days of close monitoring for signs of heart failure is recommended.
- Prophylactic diuretics and ACE inhibitors may be indicated in high-risk patients.
- A routine echocardiographic examination post-delivery in high-risk women is advisable, paying careful attention to the aortic root in women with Marfan syndrome or aortic valve disease.
-The risk of thrombo-embolic complications is further increased post-partum and anticoagulation should be adjusted accordingly.

**For heart failure and with normal ventricular function,**

-a short observation period of several hours up to 48 h post-partum might be sufficient.

Lactation is possible in most women with heart disease; it might be contraindicated due to medication use, severely decreased effort tolerance, or risk of mastitis and bacteremia in some women. The use of diuretics can complicate the initiation of milk production.

# 62  Extremely Premature Babies between22and26weeks Gestation

## 62.1   Action in Established Pre-term Labour pathway

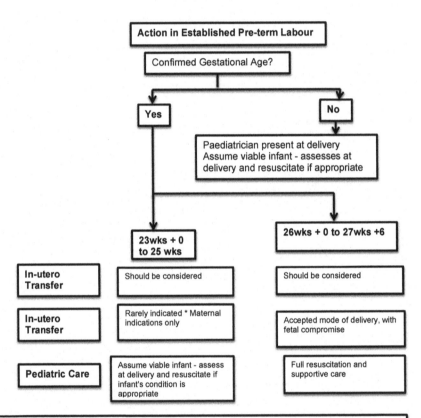

**Action in Established Pre-term Labour**

Confirmed Gestational Age?

**Yes**

**No**

Paediatrician present at delivery
Assume viable infant - assesses at
delivery and resuscitate if appropriate

**23wks + 0
to 25 wks**

**26wks + 0 to 27wks +6**

| **In-utero Transfer** | Should be considered | Should be considered |
| **In-utero Transfer** | Rarely indicated * Maternal indications only | Accepted mode of delivery, with fetal compromise |
| **Pediatric Care** | Assume viable infant - assess at delivery and resuscitate if infant's condition is appropriate | Full resuscitation and supportive care |

Here are wide variations in prognosis &outcome for infants born between 23 to 25 +6 weeks.
The management of the infant should be consistent with parents' wishes if fetal weight >= 500

# 63 Late inter-uterine death and still birth

# 63.1 Definition

## Definition

Delivery of a fetus with no signs of life known to have died after 24 completed weeks of gestation.

# 63.2 Diagnosis

## Diagnosis

**The diagnosis**
-confirmed by ultrasound
-If patient wishes repeat USS should be offered by An appropriately trained person

**Secondary features of IUD include**
- Collapse of fetal skull and overlapping bones (Spalding's sign) - Maceration resulting in unrecognizable tissue
- Hydrops
- Intra foetal gas

**Auscultation and CTG are unreliable an should not be used for diagnosis intra utrine fetal death**

# 63.3   Communication

Communication

Parents should be told in the appropriate surroundings in an expert train person in breaking bad news .If alone, offer to call partner, family or friends   Parents may need time to absorb any information

# 63.4   Isoimmunisation prevention

Isoimmunisation prevention

-Identify the patient blood group and Rh status

-if the patient Rh negative do Kleihauer testing

-administered anti D if needed within 72 hrs (can be given up to 10 days )

## 63.5   Mode of delivery and timing

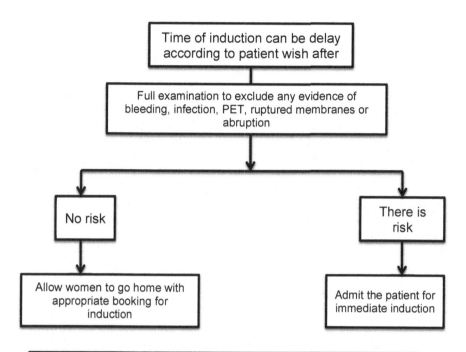

If delayed > 48 hours the mother should be monitored for evidence of DIC twice weekly

# 63.6 Mode of delivery

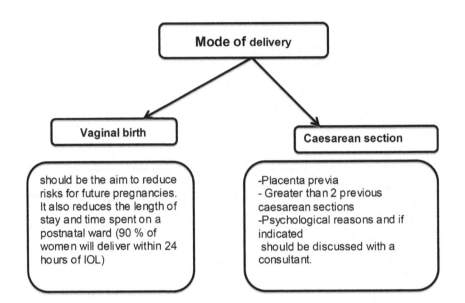

Mode of delivery

Vaginal birth

should be the aim to reduce risks for future pregnancies. It also reduces the length of stay and time spent on a postnatal ward (90 % of women will deliver within 24 hours of IOL)

Caesarean section

-Placenta previa
- Greater than 2 previous caesarean sections
-Psychological reasons and if indicated
 should be discussed with a consultant.

# 63.7 IOL see flowchart

IOL in IUFD

A combination of mifepristone and prostaglandin preparation should usually be recommended

Day 1: oral 200mg Mifepristone
Day 3: PV (break tablets in half) 100mcg 4hrly X 4 doses.

Prostaglandin induction
See the flow chart

-Syntocinon augmentation should be a consultant decision

-**DO NOT** rupture membranes to prevent chorioamnitis

-If previous uterine scar case discussed with consultant induction of labou according to flow chart
Women with 2 previous LSCS should be advised that in general the absolute risk of IOL with prostaglandin is only a little higher than for a women with single previous scar.   Women with > 2 LSCS or atypical scars should be advised that the safety is unknown
**Misoprostol can be used in preference to PG E2 due to its equivalent safety and efficiency with lower cost.**

## Antibiotics

Prophylaxis for GBS is not required if patient is known to be GBS
Antibiotics are not required unless there is evidence of infection

## Thromboprophylaxis

Standard prophylaxis guidelines should be followed IUD is not a risk factor

## Suppression of lactation

-Good breast support  Ice packs  NSAIDS
- Pharmacological suppression Cabergoline is superior to bromocriptine.
  Cabergoline is an ergot derivative; it should not be used if there is a
history of PET or a strong F/H of CVS disease or thromboembolic disease

1mg Carbergoline STAT during the first day post partum before lactation
begins 250mcg 12 hourly for two days

if lactation has begun  Bromocriptine (2.5mg BD) X 14 days.

# 63.8   Investigations

Investigations

Necessity of investigation should be explain th the cobbles . Following should be considered: CBC

-Kleihauer test   Blood group and antibody screen

  Coagulation and fibrinogen (abruption, DIC)

HbA1C if known diabetes, random blood glucose if not

Urea and Electrolytes   Liver function tests   Bile acids

TFT's (occult thyroid disease)

CRP, Blood cultures (sepsis)

Syphilis / Parvovirus / CMV / Toxoplasmosis / Rubella serology

Urine culture

High vaginal swab   Cervical swabs   Placental swab   Placental histology

Fetal blood for culture   Fetal skin swabs for culture   Fetal skin biopsy / placental biopsy for karyotyping (NOT FIXED IN FORMALIN) Post mortem

# 64 Obstetric temple

## 64.1 Temple of vacuum delivery

## 64.2 Temple of forceps delivery

## 64.3 Temple of shoulder dystocia

**Temple of vacuum delivery**

**Consent sign by patient**

Name of obstetrician conducting the delivery ----------------------

title ---------------------

G------P------

PA head engagement ---------    Fetal size ----------

Contraction ring       yes    no

Bladder evacuated      yes    no

**Vaginal examination**

Cervix -----------

Vertex station ------------

Patient on syntocinon      yes    no

                Time h: m successful?

  Application time: _____: _____

Traction start time: _____: _____

     Delivery time: _____: _____

# of pulls: _____

# Of pop-offs:--------------

Time announce failed vacuum --------

**Delivery accomplished by:**

__ Spontaneous vaginal delivery

__ Forceps (assisted vaginal delivery)

__ Cesarean delivery

Time for the baby delivery       Baby A/S

Name of pediatrician attending the delivery

Title ---------------------

Time of call for pediatrician -----------

Time of arrival of pediatrician -----------

Baby umbilical arterial cord ph------ BD------co2------Hco3------

Baby umbilical venous cord ph------- BD-------co2-----Hco3------

**Development of complication**

Perineal laceration -------

3$^{rd}$ or 4$^{th}$ degree perineal tear -------------

Post partum Haemorrhage---------

Shoulder dystocia ------------

Any other complication -------------------

Time of delivery of placenta -----------

**Comment :**

---

**Was delivery vacuum extraction ?**

Yes__ No__

**If no, why?**

__ Failure of descent

__Equipment failure

__ Fetal intolerance

__ Maternal intolerance

**Temple of forceps delivery**

**Consent sign by patient**

Name of obstetrician conducting the delivery ------------------------

title ----------------------

G------P------

PA head engagement ----------  Fetal size -----------

Contraction ring  yes  no

Bladder evacuated  yes  no

**Vaginal examination**

Cervix -----------------

Vertex station -------------

Patient on syntocinon  yes  no

Time h: m

Application time: _____: _____

Traction start time: _____: _____

Delivery time: _____: _____

# of pulls: _____

**Delivery accomplished by**

__ Spontaneous vaginal delivery

__ forceps delivery

__ Cesarean delivery

Time for the baby delivery  Baby A/S

Name of pediatrician attending the delivery

Title --------------------

Time of call for pediatrician -----------

Time of arrival of pediatrician -----------

Baby umbilical arterial cord ph------- BD-------co2-------Hco3------

Baby umbilical venous cord ph------- BD-------co2-----Hco3------

**Development of complication**

Perineal laceration ------

$3^{rd}$ or $4^{th}$ degree perineal tear ---------------

Post partum Haemorrhage----------

Shoulder dystocia ----------

Any other complication --------------------

Time of delivery of placenta -----------

Comment

---

**Application**

Easy__ Moderate__ Difficult __

**Rotation:**

N/A __ Easy __ Moderate __ Difficult__

**Traction**

Easy __ Moderate __ Difficult__

**Temple of shoulder dystocia**

Name of midwife conducting the delivery --------------------

Name of obstetrician conducting the delivery

title ---------------------

G------P-------

PA head engagement ----------           Fetal size ----------

Shoulder dystocia anticipated           yes        no

Bladder evacuated           yes        no

**Vaginal examination**

Cervix --------------

Vertex station ------------

Patient on syntocinon           yes        no

Time of announce call for help

Time for arrival of obstetrician ---------

Name of obstetrician

Title ---------------------

Time for the **MCROBERT's** maneuver

Time for the Anterior shoulder disimpaction

Time for the Wood Screw manoeuver

Time for deliver by posterior arm

Time for proceeds for Deliver posterior arm delivery

Proceeded for ceaserian section Zavenelli/symphisiotomy/cleidotomy

Time for the baby delivery

Baby A/S

Name of pediatrician attending the delivery

Title ------------------------

Time of call for pediatrician ------------

Time of arrival of pediatrician -----------

Baby umbilical arterial cord ph------ BD------$CO_2$------Hco3------

Baby umbilical venous cord ph------ BD-------$CO_2$------Hco3------

**Development of complication**

Perineal laceration -------

3$^{rd}$ or 4$^{th}$ degree perineal tear --------------

Post partum Haemorrhage----------

Neurological defecate ------------

Any other complication -------------------

Time of delivery of placenta -----------

Comment

# 65  Reference

## 65.1  chapter 1 reference

1. NICE 2008Antenatal care for uncomplicated pregnancies Clinical guideline Published: 26 March 2008 Nice.org.uk/guidance/cg62
2. World Health Organization 2016 WHO recommendations on antenatal care for a positive pregnancy experience. I.World Health Organization.

## 65.2  chapter 2 reference

1. Deaton JL, Honoré GM, Huffman CS, Bauguess P. Early transvaginal ultrasound following an accurately dated pregnancy: the importance of finding a yolk sac or fetal heart motion. Hum Reprod 1997; 12:2820.
2. Nybo Andersen AM, Wohlfahrt J, Christens P, et al. Maternal age and fetal loss: population based register linkage study. BMJ 2000; 320:1708.
3. Savaris RF, de Moraes GS, Cristovam RA, Braun RD. Are antibiotics necessary after 48 hours of improvement in infected/septic abortions? A randomized controlled trial followed by a cohort study. Am J Obstet Gynecol 2011; 204:301.e1.
4. Sawaya GF, Grady D, Kerlikowske K, Grimes DA. Antibiotics at the time of induced abortion: the case for universal prophylaxis based on a meta-analysis. Obstet Gynecol 1996; 87:884.
5. Grossman D, Blanchard K, Blumenthal P. Complications after second trimester surgical and medical abortion. Reprod Health Matters 2008; 16:173.

# 65.3   chapter 3 referance

Reference
1. Boehlen F, Hohlfeld P, Extermann P, et al. Platelet count at term pregnancy: a reappraisal of the threshold. Obstet Gynecol 2000; 95:29.
2. Neunert C, Lim W, Crowther M, et al. The American Society of Hematology 2011 evidence-based practice guideline for immune thrombocytopenia. Blood 2011; 117:4190.
3. Gill KK, Kelton JG. Management of idiopathic thrombocytopenic purpura in pregnancy. Semin Hematol 2000; 37:275.
4. Webert KE, Mittal R, Sigouin C, et al. A retrospective 11-year analysis of obstetric patients with idiopathic thrombocytopenic purpura. Blood 2003; 102:4306.
5. Chong BH. Primary immune thrombocytopenia: understanding pathogenesis is the key to better treatments. J Thromb Haemost 2009; 7:319
6. Koyama S, Tomimatsu T, Kanagawa T, et al. Reliable predictors of neonatal immune thrombocytopenia in pregnant women with idiopathic thrombocytopenic purpura. Am J Hematol 2012; 87:15.
7. Allford SL, Hunt BJ, Rose P, et al. Guidelines on the diagnosis and management of the thrombotic microangiopathic haemolytic anaemias. Br J Haematol 2003; 120:556.
8. McMinn JR, George JN. Evaluation of women with clinically suspected thrombotic thrombocytopenic purpura-hemolytic uremic syndrome during pregnancy. J Clin Apher 2001; 16:202.
9. Webert KE, Mittal R, Sigouin C, et al. A retrospective 11-year analysis of obstetric patients with idiopathic thrombocytopenic purpura. Blood 2003; 102:4306.

## 65.4 Chapter 4 reference

1. Stephansson O, Dickman PW, Johansson A, Cnattingius S. Maternal hemoglobin concentration during pregnancy and risk of stillbirth. JAMA 2000; 284:2611.
2. Juncà J, Fernández-Avilés F, Oriol A, et al. The usefulness of the serum transferrin receptor in detecting iron deficiency in the anemia of chronic disorders. Haematologica 1998; 83:676.
3. Recommendations to prevent and control iron deficiency in the United States. Centers for Disease Control and Prevention. MMWR Morb Mortal Wkly Rep 1998; 47(RR-3):1.
4. Brugnara C. Iron deficiency and erythropoiesis: new diagnostic approaches. Clin Chem 2003; 49:1573.

## 65.5 Chapter 5 Reference

1. Moore TR. Amniotic fluid dynamics reflect fetal and maternal health and disease. Obstet Gynecol 2010; 116:759.
2. Zhu X, Jiang S, Hu Y, et al. The expression of aquaporin 8 and aquaporin 9 in fetal membranes and placenta in term pregnancies complicated by idiopathic polyhydramnios. Early Hum Dev 2010;
86:657

## 65.6 Chapter 6 Reference

1. Moore TR. Amniotic fluid dynamics reflect fetal and maternal health and disease. Obstet Gynecol 2010; 116:759.
2. Zhu X, Jiang S, Hu Y, et al. The expression of aquaporin 8 and aquaporin 9 in fetal membranes and placenta in term pregnancies complicated by idiopathic polyhydramnios. Early Hum Dev 2010;
86:657

# 65.7　chapter 7 Reference

1. Bahado-Singh RO, Kovanci E, Jeffres A, et al. The Doppler cerebroplacental ratio and perinatal outcome in intrauterine growth restriction. Am J Obstet Gynecol 1999; 180:750.
2. Chambers SE, Hoskins PR, Haddad NG, et al. A comparison of fetal abdominal circumference measurements and Doppler ultrasound in the prediction of small-for-dates babies and fetal compromise. Br J Obstet Gynaecol 1989; 96:803.
3. Ferrazzi E, Nicolini U, Kustermann A, Pardi G. Routine obstetric ultrasound: effectiveness of cross-sectional screening for fetal growth retardation. J Clin Ultrasound 1986; 14:17.
4. Zhang J, Mikolajczyk R, Grewal J, et al. Prenatal application of the individualized fetal growth reference. Am J Epidemiol 2011; 173:539.
5. Dugoff L, Lynch AM, Cioffi-Ragan D, et al. First trimester uterine artery Doppler abnormalities predict subsequent intrauterine growth restriction. Am J Obstet Gynecol 2005; 193:1208.
6. Vasconcelos RP, Brazil Frota Aragão JR, Costa Carvalho FH, et al. Differences in neonatal outcome in fetuses with absent versus reverse end-diastolic flow in umbilical artery Doppler. Fetal Diagn Ther 2010; 28:160.
7. Nozaki AM, Francisco RP, Fonseca ES, et al. Fetal hemodynamic changes following maternal betamethasone administration in pregnancies with fetal growth restriction and absent end-diastolic flow in the umbilical artery. Acta Obstet Gynecol Scand 2009; 88:350.

## 65.8 Chapter 8 Reference

1. Delzell JE Jr, Lefevre ML. Urinary tract infections during pregnancy. Am Fam Physician 2000; 61:713.
2. Nicolle LE, Bradley S, Colgan R, et al. Infectious Diseases Society of America guidelines for the diagnosis and treatment of asymptomatic bacteriuria in adults. Clin Infect Dis 2005; 40:643.
3. Lin K, Fajardo K, U.S. Preventive Services Task Force. Screening for asymptomatic bacteriuria in adults: evidence for the U.S. Preventive Services Task Force reaffirmation recommendation statement. Ann Intern Med 2008; 149:W20.
4. Schito GC, Naber KG, Botto H, et al. The ARESC study: an international survey on the antimicrobial resistance of pathogens involved in uncomplicated urinary tract infections. Int J Antimicrob Agents 2009; 34:407.
5. Archabald KL, Friedman A, Raker CA, Anderson BL. Impact of trimester on morbidity of acute pyelonephritis in pregnancy. Am J Obstet Gynecol 2009; 201:406.e1.

## 65.9 Chapter 9 Reference

1. Gonzalez MC, Reyes H, Arrese M, et al. Intrahepatic cholestasis of pregnancy in twin pregnancies. J Hepatol 1989; 9:84.
2. Bacq Y, Sapey T, Bréchot MC, et al. Intrahepatic cholestasis of pregnancy: a French prospective study. Hepatology 1997; 26:358.
3. Pusl T, Beuers U. Intrahepatic cholestasis of pregnancy. Orphanet J Rare Dis 2007; 2:26.
4. Williamson C, Hems LM, Goulis DG, et al. Clinical outcome in a series of cases of obstetric cholestasis identified via a patient support group. BJOG 2004; 111:676.

5. Glantz A, Marschall HU, Mattsson LA. Intrahepatic cholestasis of pregnancy: relationships between bile acid levels and fetal complication rates. Hepatology 2004;40:467–74.

## 65.10   Chapter 10

1. Lamont RF, Sobel JD, Carrington D, et al. Varicella-zoster virus (chickenpox) infection in pregnancy. BJOG 2011; 118:1155.
2. Cohen A, Moschopoulos P, Maschopoulos P, et al. Congenital varicella syndrome: the evidence for secondary prevention with varicella-zoster immune globulin. CMAJ 2011; 183:204.
3. Harger JH, Ernest JM, Thurnau GR, et al. Risk factors and outcome of varicella-zoster virus pneumonia in pregnant women. J Infect Dis 2002; 185:422.
4. Centers for Disease Control and Prevention (CDC). FDA approval of an extended period for administering VariZIG for postexposure prophylaxis of varicella. MMWR Morb Mortal Wkly Rep 2012; 61:212.

## 65.11   Chapter 11 Reference

1. Bahia-Oliveira LM, Jones JL, Azevedo-Silva J, et al. Highly endemic, waterborne toxoplasmosis in north Rio de Janeiro state, Brazil. Emerg Infect Dis 2003; 9:55.
2. Gilbert RE, Freeman K, Lago EG, et al. Ocular sequelae of congenital toxoplasmosis in Brazil compared with Europe. PLoS Negl Trop Dis 2008; 2:e277.
3. Binquet C, Wallon M, Quantin C, et al. [Evaluation of prevention strategies for congenital toxoplasmosis: a critical

review of medico-economic studies]. Rev Epidemiol Sante Publique 2002; 50:475.

4. Gilbert RE, Gras L, Wallon M, et al. Effect of prenatal treatment on mother to child transmission of Toxoplasma gondii: retrospective cohort study of 554 mother-child pairs in Lyon, France. Int J Epidemiol 2001; 30:1303.

5. Flack NJ, Sepulveda W, Bower S, Fisk NM. Acute maternal hydration in third-trimester oligohydramnios: effects on amniotic fluid volume, uteroplacental perfusion, and fetal blood flow and urine output. Am J Obstet Gynecol 1995; 173:1186.

6. Brace RA. Physiology of amniotic fluid volume regulation. Clin Obstet Gynecol 1997; 40:280.

7. Magann EF, Chauhan SP, Doherty DA, et al. A review of idiopathic hydramnios and pregnancy outcomes. Obstet Gynecol Surv 2007; 62:795.

8. Kramer MS, Rouleau J, Baskett TF, et al. Amniotic-fluid embolism and medical induction of labour: a retrospective, population-based cohort study. Lancet2006; 368:1444.

# 65.12 Chapter 12 Reference

1. Centers for Disease Control and Prevention (CDC). Cephalosporin susceptibility among Neisseria gonorrhoeae isolates--United States, 2000-2010. MMWR Morb Mortal Wkly Rep 2011; 60:873.

2. file://www.cdc.gov/std/treatment/2010/default.htm (Accessed on January 13, 2011)

3. Centers for Disease Control and Prevention (CDC). Update to CDC's Sexually transmitted diseases treatment guidelines, 2010: oral cephalosporins no longer a recommended treatment for gonococcal infections. MMWR Morb Mortal Wkly Rep 2012; 61:590.

# 65.13   Chapter 13 Reference

1. Sookoian S. Liver disease during pregnancy: acute viral hepatitis. Ann Hepatol 2006; 5:231.
2. Tan HH, Lui HF, Chow WC. Chronic hepatitis B virus (HBV) infection in pregnancy. Hepatol Int 2008; 2:370.
3. Gill US, et al. Factors determining bone mineral density loss in chronic hepatitis B patients: is tenofovir disoproxil fumarate the main culprit? Gut 2011; 60:A230.
4. Hill JB, Sheffield JS, Kim MJ, et al. Risk of hepatitis B transmission in breast-fed infants of chronic hepatitis B carriers. Obstet Gynecol 2002; 99:1049.

# 65.14   Chapter 14 Reference

1. Stagno, S. Britt, W. Cytomegalovirus infections. In: Infectious Diseases of the Fetus and Newborn Infant, 6th ed, Remington, JS, Klein, JO, Wilson, CB, Baker, CJ (Eds), Elsevier Saunders, Philadelphia 2006. p.739.
2. Ross SA, Novak Z, Pati S, et al. Mixed infection and strain diversity in congenital cytomegalovirus infection. J Infect Dis 2011; 204:1003.
3. Simonazzi G, Guerra B, Bonasoni P, et al. Fetal cerebral periventricular halo at midgestation: an ultrasound finding suggestive of fetal cytomegalovirus infection. Am J Obstet Gynecol 2010; 202:599.e1.
4. Lipitz S, Hoffmann C, Feldman B, et al. Value of prenatal ultrasound and magnetic resonance imaging in assessment of congenital primary cytomegalovirus infection. Ultrasound Obstet Gynecol 2010; 36:709.

## 65.15   Chapter 15 Reference:

1. Management of genital Herpes in Pregnancy, RCOG Green-top guideline No. 30, September 2007
2. Baker DA. Management of Herpes in Pregnancy. ACOG Practice Bulletin 8. Washington, DC: American College of Obstetricians and Gynecologists, 1999.
3. Brown ZA, Wald A, Morrow RA, Selke S, Zeh J, Corey L. Effect of serologic status and cesarean delivery on transmission rate of herpes simplex virus from mother to infant. JAMA 2003;289:203–9.

## 65.16   Chapter 16 Reference

1. Miyagawa S, Takahashi Y, Nagai A, et al. Angio-oedema in a neonate with IgG antibodies to parvovirus B19 following intrauterine parvovirus B19 infection. Br J Dermatol 2000; 143:428.
2. Prospective study of human parvovirus (B19) infection in pregnancy. Public Health Laboratory Service Working Party on Fifth Disease. BMJ 1990; 300:1166.
3. Enders M, Weidner A, Rosenthal T, et al. Improved diagnosis of gestational parvovirus B19 infection at the time of nonimmune fetal hydrops. J Infect Dis 2008; 197:58.
4. Borna S, Mirzaie F, Hanthoush-Zadeh S, et al. Middle cerebral artery peak systolic velocity and ductus venosus velocity in the investigation of nonimmune hydrops. J Clin Ultrasound 2009; 37:385.

## 65.17   Chapter 17 reference

1. Rodis JF, Quinn DL, Gary GW Jr, et al. Management and outcomes of pregnancies complicated by human B19

parvovirus infection: a prospective study. Am J Obstet Gynecol 1990; 163:1168.

2. Skjöldebrand-Sparre L, Tolfvenstam T, Papadogiannakis N, et al. Parvovirus B19 infection: association with third-trimester intrauterine fetal death. BJOG 2000; 107:476.

3. Marton T, Martin WL, Whittle MJ. Hydrops fetalis and neonatal death from human parvovirus B19: an unusual complication. Prenat Diagn 2005; 25:543.

4. Cosmi E, Mari G, Delle Chiaie L, et al. Noninvasive diagnosis by Doppler ultrasonography of fetal anemia resulting from parvovirus infection. Am J Obstet Gynecol 2002; 187:1290.

## 65.18 Chapter 18 Referance

1. FIUMARA NJ. Congenital syphilis in Massachusetts. N Engl J Med 1951; 245:634.

2. Centers for Disease Control and Prevention (CDC). Congenital syphilis - United States, 2003-2008. MMWR Morb Mortal Wkly Rep 2010; 59:413.

3. U.S. Preventive Services Task Force. Screening for syphilis infection in pregnancy: U.S. Preventive Services Task Force reaffirmation recommendation statement. Ann Intern Med 2009; 150:705.

4. American College of Obstetricians and Gynecologists and American Academy of Pediatrics. Guidelines for Perinatal Care, 7th edition, 2012.

5. Yates AB. Management of patients with a history of allergy to beta-lactam antibiotics. Am J Med 2008; 121:572.

## 65.19 Chapter 19 Reference

1. Phylipsen M, Yamsri S, Treffers EE, et al. Non-invasive prenatal diagnosis of beta-thalassemia and sickle-cell

disease using pyrophosphorolysis-activated polymerization and melting curve analysis. Prenat Diagn 2012; 32:578.

2. Wang X, Seaman C, Paik M, et al. Experience with 500 prenatal diagnoses of sickle cell diseases: the effect of gestational age on affected pregnancy outcome. Prenat Diagn 1994; 14:851.

3. Martin JN Jr, Martin RW, Morrison JC. Acute management of sickle cell crisis in pregnancy. Clin Perinatol 1986; 13:853.

4. Jans SM, de Jonge A, Lagro-Janssen AL. Maternal and perinatal outcomes amongst haemoglobinopathy carriers: a systematic review. Int J Clin Pract 2010; 64:1688.

5. Winder AD, Johnson S, Murphy J, Ehsanipoor RM. Epidural analgesia for treatment of a sickle cell crisis during pregnancy. Obstet Gynecol 2011; 118:495.

# 65.20   Chapter 20 Reference

1. Yamazaki K, Sato K, Shizume K, et al. Potent thyrotropic activity of human chorionic gonadotropin variants in terms of 125I incorporation and de novo synthesized thyroid hormone release in human thyroid follicles. J Clin Endocrinol Metab 1995; 80:473.

2. Bajoria R, Fisk NM. Permeability of human placenta and fetal membranes to thyrotropin-stimulating hormone in vitro. Pediatr Res 1998; 43:621.

3. Stagnaro-Green A, Abalovich M, Alexander E, et al. Guidelines of the American Thyroid Association for the diagnosis and management of thyroid disease during pregnancy and postpartum. Thyroid 2011; 21:1081.

4. Idris I, Srinivasan R, Simm A, Page RC. Maternal hypothyroidism in early and late gestation: effects on neonatal and obstetric outcome. Clin Endocrinol (Oxf) 2005; 63:560.

5. hangaratinam S, Tan A, Knox E, et al. Association between thyroid autoantibodies and miscarriage and preterm birth: meta-analysis of evidence. BMJ 2011; 342:d2616.

6. Azizi F, Khoshniat M, Bahrainian M, Hedayati M. Thyroid function and intellectual development of infants nursed by mothers taking methimazole. J Clin Endocrinol Metab 2000; 85:3233.

7. Huel C, Guibourdenche J, Vuillard E, et al. Use of ultrasound to distinguish between fetal hyperthyroidism and hypothyroidism on discovery of a goiter. Ultrasound Obstet Gynecol 2009; 33:412.

# 65.21 Chapter 21 Reference

1. Metzger BE, Coustan DR (Eds.): Proceed- ings of the Fourth International Work- shop-Conference on Gestational Diabetes Mellitus. Diabetes Care 21 (Suppl. 2):B1– B167, 1998

2. International Association of Diabetes and Pregnancy Study Groups Consensus Panel, Metzger BE, Gabbe SG, Persson B, Buchanan TA, Catalano PA, Damm P, et al. International association of diabetes and pregnancy study groups recommendations on the diagnosis and classification of hyperglycemia in pregnancy. Diabetes Care 2010;33:676–82.

3. Kim C, Liu T, Valdez R, Beckles GL. Does frank diabetes in first-degree relatives of a pregnant woman affect the likelihood of her developing gestational diabetes mellitus or nongestational diabetes? Am J Obstet Gynecol 2009; 201:576.e1.

4. Lowe LP, Metzger BE, Dyer AR, et al. Hyperglycemia and Adverse Pregnancy Outcome (HAPO) Study: associations of maternal A1C and glucose with pregnancy outcomes. Diabetes Care 2012; 35:574.

5. 30. Landon MB, Mele L, Spong CY, et al. The relationship between maternal glycemia and perinatal outcome. Obstet Gynecol 2011; 117:218.
6. 10. Han S, Crowther, CA, et al. Different types of dietary advice for women with gestational diabetes mellitus. Cochrane Database Syst Rev 2013; :CD009275.
7. Metzger BE, Ravnikar V, Vileisis RA, Freinkel N. "Accelerated starvation" and the skipped breakfast in late normal pregnancy. Lancet 1982; 1:588.
8. Rizzo T, Metzger BE, Burns WJ, Burns K. Correlations between antepartum maternal metabolism and child intelligence. N Engl J Med 1991; 325:911.

# 65.22 Chapter 22 Reference

1. Wier LM, Witt E, Burgess J, Elixhauser A. A Healthcare Cost and Utilization Project. Statistical Brief 102. Hospitalizations Related to Diabetes in Pregnancy 2008, Agency for Health Care Policy and Research, Rockville, MD. 2010.
2. Ehrlich SF, Crites YM, Hedderson MM, et al. The risk of large for gestational age across increasing categories of pregnancy glycemia. Am J Obstet Gynecol 2011; 204:240. e1.
3. Holmes VA, Young IS, Patterson CC, et al. Optimal glycemic control, pre-eclampsia, and gestational hypertension in women with type 1 diabetes in the diabetes and pre-eclampsia intervention trial. Diabetes Care 2011; 34:1683.
4. NICE 2015.

# 65.23 Chapter 23 Reference

1. Sibai BM. Chronic hypertension in pregnancy. Obstet Gynecol 2002; 100:369–77.

2. Executive summary: hypertension in pregnancy. American Col- lege of Obstetricians and Gynecologists. Obstet Gynecol 2013; 122:1122–31.
3. Bujold E, Roberge S, Lacasse Y et al. (2010) Prevention of preeclampsia and intrauterine growth restriction with aspirin started in early pregnancy. Obstetrics & Gynecology 116: 402–12 abstract: www.greenjournal/Abstract/2010/08000
4. Hypertension in pregnancy: Evidence update May2012

## 65.24   Chapter 25 Reference

1. Mintz G, Niz J, Gutierrez G, et al. Prospective study of pregnancy in systemic lupus erythematosus. Results of a multidisciplinary approach. J Rheumatol 1986; 13:732.
2. Ruiz-Irastorza G, Khamashta MA. Lupus and pregnancy: ten questions and some answers. Lupus 2008; 17:416.
3. Kong NC. Pregnancy of a lupus patient--a challenge to the nephrologist. Nephrol Dial Transplant 2006; 21:268.
4. Chakravarty EF, Colón I, Langen ES, et al. Factors that predict prematurity and preeclampsia in pregnancies that are complicated by systemic lupus erythematosus. Am J Obstet Gynecol 2005;
5. Andrade R, Sanchez ML, Alarcón GS, et al. Adverse pregnancy outcomes in women with systemic lupus erythematosus from a multiethnic US cohort: LUMINA (LVI) [corrected]. Clin Exp Rheumatol 2008; 26:268.
6. Ross G, Sammaritano L, Nass R, Lockshin M. Effects of mothers' autoimmune disease during pregnancy on learning disabilities and hand preference in their children. Arch Pediatr Adolesc Med 2003; 157:397.
7. Izmirly PM, Costedoat-Chalumeau N, Pisoni CN, et al. Maternal use of hydroxychloroquine is associated with a reduced risk of recurrent anti-SSA/Ro-antibody-associated

cardiac manifestations of neonatal lupus. Circulation 2012; 126:76.

8. Lockshin MD, Sammaritano LR. Lupus pregnancy. Autoimmunity 2003; 36:33.

9. Andrade RM, McGwin G Jr, Alarcón GS, et al. Predictors of post-partum damage accrual in systemic lupus erythematosus: data from LUMINA, a multiethnic US cohort (XXXVIII). Rheumatology (Oxford) 2006; 45:1380.

10. Al-Herz A, Schulzer M, Esdaile JM. Survey of antimalarial use in lupus pregnancy and lactation. J Rheumatol 2002; 29:700.

## 65.25   Chapter 26 reference

1. Bar J, Ben-Rafael Z, Padoa A, et al. Prediction of pregnancy outcome in subgroups of women with renal disease. Clin Nephrol 2000; 53:437.

2. Imbasciati E, Gregorini G, Cabiddu G, et al. Pregnancy in CKD stages 3 to 5: fetal and maternal outcomes. Am J Kidney Dis 2007; 49:753.

3. Piccoli GB, Conijn A, Consiglio V, et al. Pregnancy in dialysis patients: is the evidence strong enough to lead us to change our counseling policy? Clin J Am Soc Nephrol 2010; 5:62.

## 65.26   Chapter 27 Reference

1. Royal College of Obstetricians and Gynaecologist. Green top guidelines. Anti-D immunoglobulin for Rh prophylaxis. RCOG, London, 2002.

2. Silva, M (Ed). Standards for blood banks and transfusion services. 24th ed. American Association of Blood Banks. Amercian Association of Blood Banks, Bethesda, MD, 2006

3. Kumpel BM. Analysis of factors affecting quantification of fetomaternal hemorrhage by flow cytometry. Transfusion 2000; 40:1376.
4. Lafferty J, Raby A, Keeney M, et al. Inaccurate doses of Rh immune globulin after Rh-incompatible fetomaternal hemorrhage-survey of laboratory practice. Arch Pathol Lab Med 2009; 133:1910.
5. Sandler SG, Gottschall JL. Postpartum Rh immunoprophylaxis. Obstet Gynecol 2012; 120:1428.
6. Wagner FF, Gassner C, Müller TH, et al. Molecular basis of weak D phenotypes. Blood 1999; 93:385.
7. Flegel WA. Molecular genetics and clinical applications for RH. Transfus Apher Sci 2011; 44:81

# 65.27   Chapter 28 Reference

1. Sabers A. Influences on seizure activity in pregnant women with epilepsy. Epilepsy Behav 2009; 15:230.
2. Morrow JI, Hunt SJ, Russell AJ, et al. Folic acid use and major congenital malformations in offspring of women with epilepsy: a prospective study from the UK Epilepsy and Pregnancy Register. J Neurol Neurosurg Psychiatry 2009; 80:506.
3. AAN guideline summary for clinicians. Management issues for women with epilepsy. www.aan.com/professionals/practice/pdfs/women_epilepsy.pdf (Accessed on March 7, 2005).
4. Meador KJ, Baker GA, Browning N, et al. Effects of breastfeeding in children of women taking antiepileptic drugs. Neurology 2010; 75:1954.

## 65.28   Chapter 29 Reference

1. Drenthen W, Pieper PG, Roos-Hesselink JW, et al. Outcome of pregnancy in women with congenital heart disease: a literature review. J Am Coll Cardiol 2007; 49:2303.
2. ACOG Committee on Practice Bulletins. ACOG Practice Bulletin No. 74. Antibiotic prophylaxis for gynecologic procedures. Obstet Gynecol 2006; 108:225.
3. Elkayam U, Bitar F. Valvular heart disease and pregnancy part I: native valves. J Am Coll Cardiol 2005; 46:223.
4. Siu SC, Sermer M, Colman JM, et al. Prospective multicenter study of pregnancy outcomes in women with heart disease. Circulation 2001; 104:515.

## 65.29   Reference Section II
## Instruction manual in Labour room

1. Analgesia, anesthesia and pregnancy: a practical guide. Cambridge. 2007.
2. Antenatal Corticosteroids to Prevent Respiratory Distress Syndrome RCOG
3. Arad I. "Vacuum extraction at caesarean section neonatal outcome" J. Perinat. Med. 14 1986; 14: 137-140.
4. Best Practice in Labour and Delivery. Warren, Arulkumaran. Cambridge 2010.
5. 'Birth after previous caesarean birth' Green top guideline No45 RCOG 2007
6. Caesarean section or vaginal delivery at 24 to 28 weeks gestation:
comparison of survival and neonatal and two-year morbidity. Kitchen W, Ford GW, Doyle LW, Rickards AL, Lissenden JV, Pepperell RH, Duke JE Obstet Gynecol 1985 Aug 66:2 149-157.

7.  Changing prognosis for babies of less than 28 weeks gestation in the north of England between 1983 and 1994. Northern Neonatal Network. Tin W,Wariyar U, Hey E BMJ 1997 Jan 11;314 (7074): 107-11.

8.  Child Fetal Neonatal Ed 1996 May 74:3 F214-8.

9.  Fasubaa et al. Delivery of the impacted head of the fetus at caesarean section after prolonged obstructed labour: a randomised comparative study of two methods. Journal of Obstetrics and Gynaecology, 2002 Jul;22(4):375-378.

10. Flamm BL, Goings JR, Fuelberth N-J et al (1987) Oxytocin during labour after previous caesarean section: results of a multi-centre study. Obstetrics & Gynaecology 70: 709-12

11. Intrapartum Care for the MRCOG and beyond. RCOG Press.

12. Green–top Guideline No. 42

13. Green–top Guideline No. 56 January 2011

14. Journal of Perinatal Medicine, 2004, 32:465-469

15. K Clift & J Clift Uterine relaxation during caesarean section under regional anaesthesia: a survey of UK obstetric anaesthetists Int J or Obstet Anaesthesia.Oct 2008;17(4),374-375

16. Landesman, R, Graber, EA. Abdominovaginal delivery: modification of the cesarean section operation to facilitate delivery of the impacted head. Am J Obstet Gynecol 1984; 148:707.

17. Lydon-Rochelle M et al 2001: Risk of uterine rupture during labour among women with a prior Caesarean delivery New England Journal of Medicine 345(1):3-8

18. MacKenzie IZ, Bradley S, Embrey MP. (1984) Vaginal prostaglandins and labour induction for patients previously delivered by caesarean section. BJOG 91: 7-10

19. Management of Breech Presentation, RCOG Green-top guideline No 20B, December 2006

20. Management of genital Herpes in Pregnancy, RCOG Green-top guideline No. 30, September 2007

21. Meehan FP, Rafla NM, Burke G (1990) Regional epidural analgesia for labour following previous caesarean section. J.Obst.Gynaecol. 10: 312-6

22. Morton SC, Williams MS, Keeler EB et al Effect of epidural analgesia for labour on the caesarean delivery rate. Obstetr. Gynaecol. 1994 83(6): 1045-52

23. Nakano R. "Use of the vacuum extractor for delivery of the fetal head at caesarean section" Obstet. Gynecol.

24. NICE guidelines [CG190] Published date: December 2014

25. NICE guidelines [CG190] Published date: December 2014

26. NICE Guideline Caesarean Section Guideline 13 2004

27. NICE guideline Intrapartum Care 2007

28. Perinatal management at the lower limit of viability. JM Rennie Arch Dis

29. Prevention of Perinatal Group B Streptococcal Disease CDC, 2010

30. Saving Mothers Lives the seventh report of the Confidential Enquiries into Maternal Deaths in the United Kingdom. CEMACH London: December 2007

31. SOGC Guidelines for Vaginal Birth After Previous Caesarean Birth No 155 Feb 2005

32. Solomons E. "Delivery of the head by Malmstrom vacuum extractor during caesarean section" Obstet. Gynecol 1962; 19: 201.

33. Oxford specialist handbooks in anesthesia: Obstetric Anesthesia. Oxford. 2008.

34. Withholding or withdrawing Life Saving Treatment in Children – A Framework for Practice. Royal College of Paediatrics and Child Health, September 1997.